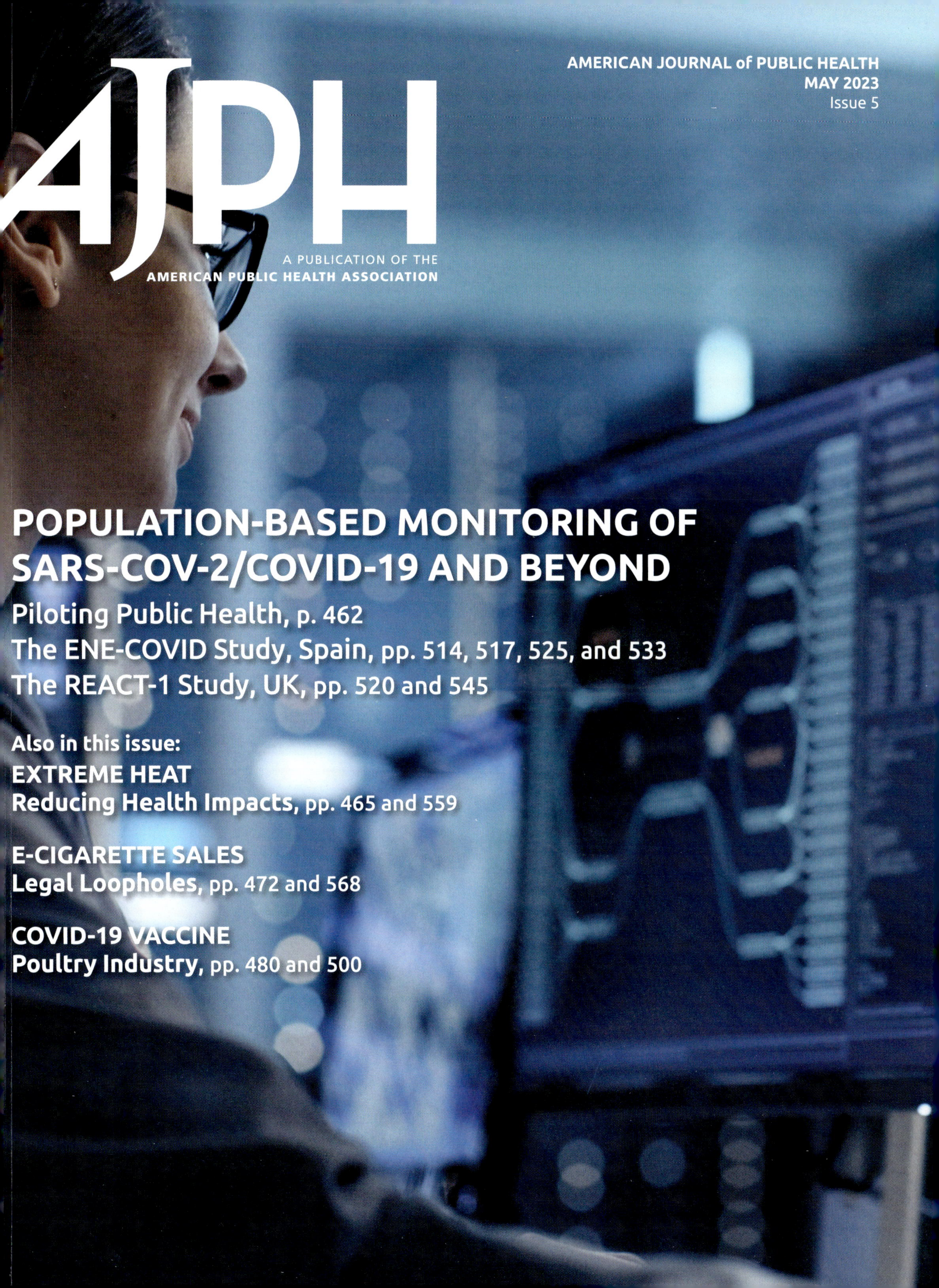

AJPH

A PUBLICATION OF THE
AMERICAN PUBLIC HEALTH ASSOCIATION

AMERICAN JOURNAL of PUBLIC HEALTH
MAY 2023
Issue 5

POPULATION-BASED MONITORING OF SARS-COV-2/COVID-19 AND BEYOND

Piloting Public Health, p. 462
The ENE-COVID Study, Spain, pp. 514, 517, 525, and 533
The REACT-1 Study, UK, pp. 520 and 545

Also in this issue:

EXTREME HEAT
Reducing Health Impacts, pp. 465 and 559

E-CIGARETTE SALES
Legal Loopholes, pp. 472 and 568

COVID-19 VACCINE
Poultry Industry, pp. 480 and 500

APHA
AMERICAN PUBLIC HEALTH ASSOCIATION
For science. For action. For health.

AJPH®, published monthly, is the official Journal of the American Public Health Association®, 800 I St NW, Washington, DC 20001-3710; (202) 777- APHA; TDD (202) 777-2500. APHA is a nongovernmental professional society founded in 1872, representing all disciplines and specialties in public health.

The *American Journal of Public Health*® (*AJPH*) (print ISSN: 0090-0036; electronic ISSN: 1541- 0048), first published in 1911, is the official journal of the American Public Health Association® (APHA). The oldest and largest organization of public health professionals in the world, APHA represents approximately 30 000 members from more than 50 occupations of public health.

Submissions: Visit www.editorialmanager.com/ajph or ajph.edmgr.com for online manuscript preparation and submission guidelines. Contributions of original unpublished research, social science analyses, scholarly essays, critical commentaries, departments, and letters to the editor are welcome. Questions? Write ajph.submissions@apha.org or call APHA at (202) 777-2469.

Print plus online subscriptions: Institutional price (print copy with online access for a single institution and all authorized users, regardless of geographic location) varies by size of organization and ranges from $993–$1445 for US organizations, and $1073–$1526 for international organizations (air delivery); multiple campuses not permitted without special arrangement. Details of the tiered pricing system at https://subscriptionoffice.com/pages/apha-landing-page. To order, write apha.subscriptions@apha.org.

Online only subscriptions: Institutional price for one institution and its authorized users (regardless of geographic location) is $878–$1307. To order, write apha.subscriptions@apha.org. For academic consortia or multisite corporate subscriptions, contact apha.subscriptions@apha.org.

Print-only subscriptions: Institutional price is US $701, $782 international.

Back print issues: A limited number of print issues are for sale. Single copies are US $49, $55 international (air delivery). Shipping included; prepay only. To order, write apha.subscriptions@apha.org.

Reprints: For prices and ordering information on 50 or more reprints, check the Reprints section at www.ajph.org. To order smaller quantities of reprints (rush delivery), use the "Purchase Article" link on the article site itself.

Electronic access: Online articles more than 10 years old are available free for personal use at www.ajph.org. Recent articles are available through pay-per-view: single PDF article for $24, single issue access for 24 hours for $33, or entire site access for 24 hours for $38.

Postal information: Periodicals postage paid at Washington, DC, and additional mailing offices. Postmaster: Send address changes to American Journal of Public Health, 800 I St NW, Washington, DC 20001-3710.

Address changes: Send to AJPH, Membership Department (members) or AJPH Subscriptions (subscribers), APHA, 800 I St NW, Washington, DC 20001-3710. Or write to membership.mail@apha. org (members) or apha.subscriptions@apha.org (subscribers).

Advertising: For pricing and other information, see www.ajph.org. Please write to ashell.alston@apha.org or call (202) 777-2470 for other advertising opportunities. Ask about special exhibit packages and sponsorships. Acceptance of advertising by the *Journal* does not imply endorsement of products.

Indexes: Publications that index or abstract articles from AJPH include the following: Ageline, Assia (Applied Social Science Index and Abstracts), Biological Abstracts, Chemical Abstracts, CINAHL, Criminal Justice Abstracts, EMBASE, EMCare, Environmental Abstracts, e-psyche, ERIC, ETOH (Alcohol and Alcohol Problems Science Database), Excerpta Medica, Food Science and Technology, General Science Index, Grateful Med, Hospital Literature Index, Human Resources Abstracts, International Pharmaceutical Abstracts (IPA), Medline, Physical Education Index, Pollution Abstracts, Psychological Abstracts, PsychINFO, Safety Science Abstracts, Sage Family Studies Abstracts, Sage Human Resources Abstracts, Science Citation Index, SCOPUS, SIIC Data Bases, Social Work Research and Abstracts, and Statistical Reference Index (SRI)/LexisNexis.

AJPH
A PUBLICATION OF THE
AMERICAN PUBLIC HEALTH ASSOCIATION

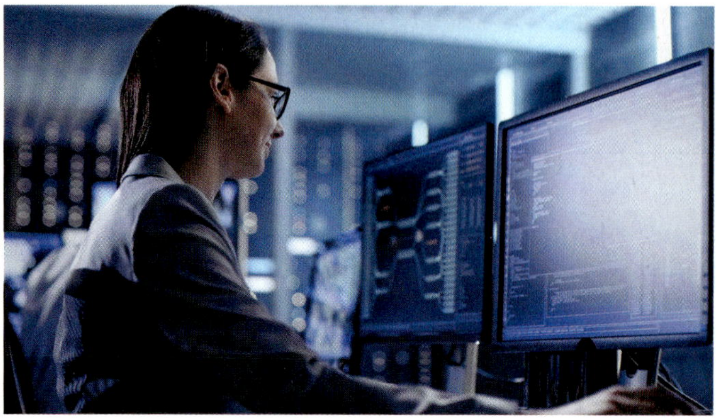

COVER: This issue of the *AJPH* explores the value of population-based information based on random samples of the population when monitoring COVID-19 and beyond. Does high resolution surveillance data translate to better projections? Do policymakers need or even use this information? What is the best way to monitor disease trajectory that will help avoid future catastrophe and result, ultimately, in healthier populations?

Cover concept and selection by Aleisha Kropf. Image by gorodenkoff. Printed with permission.

APHA
AMERICAN PUBLIC HEALTH ASSOCIATION
For science. For action. For health.

Promoting public health research, policy, practice, and education is the *AJPH* mission. As we widen our scope to embrace global issues, we also sharpen our focus to support the needs of public health practitioners. We invite contributions of original unpublished research, opinion and commentary, and letters to the editor.

The *Journal* is printed on acid-free recycled paper.

EDITOR-IN-CHIEF
Alfredo Morabia, MD, PhD

SENIOR DEPUTY EDITOR
Michael C. Costanza, PhD

DEPUTY EDITOR
Farzana Kapadia, PhD

DEPUTY STATISTICAL EDITOR
Hua He, PhD

DEPUTY EDITOR FOR OPEN ACCESS SUPPLEMENTS
Steven C. Fiala, MPH

IMAGE EDITOR
Aleisha Kropf

ASSISTANT EDITOR
Erica J. Carter, BS

STUDENT EDITOR
Michelle Sarah Livings, MPH

EDITORS
Luisa Borrell, DDS, PhD
Lisa Bowleg, PhD, MA
Theodore M. Brown, PhD
Nabarun Dasgupta, PhD, MPH
Paul C. Erwin, MD, DrPH
Laura Ferguson, PhD, MSc, MA
Daniel M. Fox, PhD
Colleen Grogan, PhD
Robert J. Kim-Farley, MD, MPH
Stewart J. Landers, JD, MCP
Tanya Telfair LeBlanc, PhD
Jonathan I. Levy, ScD
Jihong Liu, ScD
Evan Mayo-Wilson, DPhil
Marian Moser Jones, PhD, MPH
Wendy Parmet, JD
Kenneth Rochel de Camargo Jr, MD, PhD
Roger Vaughan, DrPH, MS
Eric R. Walsh-Buhi, PhD, MPH

EDITORIAL BOARD
Moya L. Alfonso, PhD, MSPH (2024)
Heather M. Brandt, PhD (2023), Chair
Amy Hagopian, PhD, MHA (2024), Vice Chair
Michael T. Halpern, MD, PhD, MPH (2024)
Kenneth Hoekstra, PhD (2024)
Amar Kanekar, PhD, MPH, MB (2023)
Shawn M. Kneipp, PhD, RN, ANP (2024)
Laura A. Nabors, PhD, MA (2024)
A.G. Palladino, MPH, MJ, MS (2023)
Laura Schwab Reese, PhD, MA (2023)
Gulzar H. Shah, PhD, MStat, MS (2024)
Mark A. Strand, PhD, MS (2023)
Joseph Telfair, DrPH, MSW, MPH (2024)
Cynthia Williams, PhD, MHA, PT (2025)
Samantha H. Xu, MPH (2023)

FORMER EDITORS-IN-CHIEF
Mary E. Northridge, PhD, MPH (Editor Emerita)
Mervyn Susser
Michel Ibrahim
Alfred Yankauer
George Rosen
Abel Wolman
Charles-Edward A. Winslow
Harry S. Mustard
Mazÿck Ravenel

STAFF
Georges C. Benjamin, MD
Executive Director/Publisher
Ashell Alston
Director of Publications
Brian Selzer
Deputy Director of Publications
Michael Henry
Associate Production Editor (Sr)
Avery Ferguson, MA
Associate Production Editor
Shokhari Tate, MPH
Journal Project Liaison
Katie Poe, MA
Associate Production Editor – Special Publications
Emily Dalton
Digital Publications Specialist

FREELANCE
Kelly Burch
Greg Edmondson
Aisha Jamil
Gary Norton
Michelle Quirk
Sarah Cook
Copyeditor
Aisha Jamil
Leona Selzer
Proofreader
Vanessa Sifford
Graphic Designer

OPEN ACCESS | ONLINE ONLY | PODCAST | DATA SUPPLEMENT AVAILABLE

EDITOR'S CHOICE

462 Piloting Public Health No. 2
A. Morabia

BOOKS & MEDIA

463 Smallpox Immunization in Colonial America: All Too Relevant Today
T. C. Smith

OPINIONS, IDEAS, & PRACTICE

EDITORIALS

465 Strengthening Heat Action Plans in the United States
M. Guardaro

468 Translating Hannah Stone's Patient-Centric Values to the Widest Possible Audience of Young People—In the Classroom as Well as the Clinic
E. S. More

470 Centering Patients' Voices in Artificial Intelligence–Based Telemedicine
S. A. Kraft

472 To End Youth Vaping as an On-Ramp to Addiction, Close Legal Loopholes and Rigorously Enforce the Law
M. A. Gottlieb

474 Looking Back: Intimate Partner Violence in Transgender Populations
B. Ethan Coston

477 Vladeck Redux: Our Endlessly Imperfect American Health Care System
J. E. McDonough

480 Public Health Practice and Health Equity for Vulnerable Workers: A Public Health of Consequence, May 2023
F. Kapadia

PERSPECTIVES

482 Medicaid Expansion: The Unfinished Promise of the Affordable Care Act
S. Kishore, M. Johnson, and S. Rosenbaum

484 Government Investment in the Marijuana Industry's Commercial Interests Harms Vulnerable Groups
L. Richter, R. Oster, and L. Vuolo

487 Cannabis Equity Initiatives: Progress, Problems, and Potentials
Y. Tony Yang, C. J. Berg, and S. Burris

490 Returns to Homelessness: Key Considerations for Using This Metric to Improve System Performance
J. Tsai and T. Byrne

NOTES FROM THE FIELD

495 Effectiveness of a Road Traffic Injury Prevention Intervention in Reducing Pedestrian Injuries, Barcelona, Spain, 2002–2019
K. Pérez, E. Santamariña-Rubio, J. Ferrando, M. J. López, and L. Badiella

500 Engaging the Poultry Industry to Vaccinate Vulnerable Populations, Arkansas, 2021–2022
A. Porter, P. James, and C. Cochran

504 Mpox Vaccine Interest Survey Prioritization and Data Flow: Maricopa County, Arizona, July–August 2022
B. J. Howard, J. E. Collins, R. N. Staab, S. Singh, E. Lara, M. Kretschmer, L. Rehder, A. Dellos, J. R. White, and A. P. Dale

509 Impact of a Large Healthy Start Program on Perinatal Outcomes, South Carolina, 2009–2019
J. Liu, L. Zhao, X. Zhao, E. M. Bawa, K. Alston, S. Karim, A. T. Merchant, J. Tang, and S. Wilcox

MONITORING COVID-19 AND BEYOND

514 Population Monitoring of SARS-CoV-2 Infections via Random Sampling During the COVID-19 Pandemic
P. Elliott, H. Ward, and S. Riley

517 Serological Studies and the Value of Information
N. E. Dean, D. H. Howard, and B. A. Lopman

520 Learning From COVID-19 to Improve Surveillance for Emerging Threats
D. B. Jernigan, D. George, and M. Lipsitch

523 Seroprevalence Studies Are Critical Early Pandemic Tools, and They Were Underappreciated During COVID-19
E. Bendavid

RESEARCH & ANALYSIS

MONITORING COVID-19 AND BEYOND

525 Design and Implementation of a Nationwide Population-Based Longitudinal Survey of SARS-CoV-2 Infection in Spain: The ENE-COVID Study
R. Pastor-Barriuso, B. Pérez-Gómez, J. Oteo-Iglesias, M. A. Hernán, M. Pérez-Olmeda, N. Fernández-de-Larrea, M. Molina, A. Fernández-García, M. Martín, I. Cruz, J. L. Sanmartín, J. León-Paniagua, J. F. Muñoz-Montalvo, F. Blanco, R. Yotti, and M. Pollán, on behalf of the ENE-COVID Study Group

533 SARS-CoV-2 Infection During the First and Second Pandemic Waves in Spain: the ENE–COVID Study
B. Pérez-Gómez, R. Pastor-Barriuso, N. Fernández-de-Larrea, M. A. Hernán, M. Pérez-Olmeda, J. Oteo-Iglesias, P. Fernández-Navarro, A. Fernández-García, M. Martín, I. Cruz, J. L. Sanmartín, J. León-Paniagua, J. F. Muñoz-Montalvo, F. Blanco, R. Yotti, and M. Pollán, on behalf of the ENE–COVID Study Group

545 Design and Implementation of a National SARS-CoV-2 Monitoring Program in England: REACT-1 Study
P. Elliott, M. Whitaker, D. Tang, O. Eales, N. Steyn, B. Bodinier, H. Wang, J. Elliott, C. Atchison, D. Ashby, W. Barclay, G. Taylor, A. Darzi, G. S. Cooke, H. Ward, C. A. Donnelly, S. Riley, and M. Chadeau-Hyam

CLIMATE CHANGE

555 Wildfire Threat to Inpatient Health Care Facilities in California, 2022
N. S. Bedi, C. Dresser, A. Yadav, A. Schroeder, and S. Balsari

LAW & ETHICS

559 Planning to Reduce the Health Impacts of Extreme Heat: A Content Analysis of Heat Action Plans in Local United States Jurisdictions
J. M. Randazza, J. J. Hess, A. Bostrom, C. Hartwell, Q. H. Adams, A. Nori-Sarma, K. R. Spangler, Y. Sun, K. R. Weinberger, G. A. Wellenius, and N. A. Errett

568 Loopholes for Underage Access in E-Cigarette Delivery Sales Laws, United States, 2022
S. Azagba, T. Ebling, O. T. Adekeye, M. Hall, and J. K. Jensen

PRACTICE

577 Ethics Principles for Artificial Intelligence–Based Telemedicine for Public Health
S. Tiribelli, A. Monnot, S. F. H. Shah, A. Arora, P. J. Toong, and S. Kong

BACKMATTER

ERRATA

585 Erratum In: "Living Alone and Suicide Risk in the United States, 2008–2019"

586 Erratum In: "SARS-CoV-2 Infection, Hospitalization, and Death in Vaccinated and Infected Individuals by Age Groups in Indiana, 2021–2022"

587 Erratum In: *American Journal of Public Health*, Volume 113, Issue 2

OTHER DEPARTMENTS

592 Subscription Form

Piloting Public Health No. 2

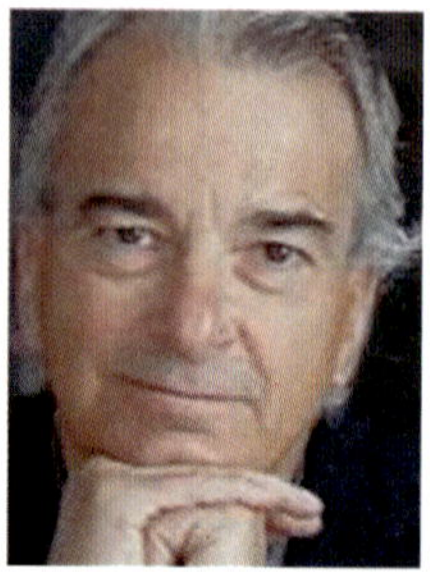

Modernizing the public health data infrastructure for the US federal government and state and local health departments is a foundational tool indispensable for piloting public health.

In this issue, we continue our exploration of the situation in the United States. As a reminder, the December 2021 issue of *AJPH* reviewed the state of the health monitoring system (https://ajph.aphapublications.org/toc/ajph/111/12). The set of reports showed that, collectively, federal, state, and city surveillance and survey programs had begun to remedy the defective structures and improved collection, processing, and dissemination plans. The system, however, was still not upgraded to provide accurate estimates of incidence and fatality rates from SARS-CoV-2 and COVID-19 and comparisons of them across time, people, and places.

The June 2022 issue of *AJPH* (https://ajph.aphapublications.org/toc/ajph/112/6) reviewed the current state of city dashboards, which have been established to remediate or complement the gaps in existing federal surveillance. These dashboards remain works in progress, needing sustainable funding and geographical integration.

The October 2022 issue (https://ajph.aphapublications.org/toc/ajph/112/10) documented the gaps in the information collected by the monitoring systems that can reveal inequities in COVID-19's impact and generate appropriate responses.

In this issue, we showcase two initiatives, one in Spain (p. 525) and the other in the United Kingdom (p. 545), that attempted to provide population-based estimates of the progression of the COVID-19 pandemic. These are, in Spain, the Seroepidemiological Survey of SARS-CoV-2 Virus Infection (*Encuesta Seroepidemiológica de la Infección por el Virus SARS-CoV-2 en España; ENE-COVID*) and, in the United Kingdom, the REal-time Assessment of Community Transmission (REACT-1) of SARS-CoV-2.

The ENE-COVID survey was nationwide, although it excluded care-home residents, hospitalized people, people in prisons, nuns and friars in convents, and residents in other collective facilities. It used two-stage sampling to randomly select households across Spanish provinces, cities, and municipalities. All residents in the household were invited to participate. The final sample included individuals of all ages. This study relied on the Spanish National Health System. Serum specimens were collected from all participants two to four weeks apart. It also provided an important observation: the prevalence of asymptomatic seropositive participants. In a companion article, Pérez-Gómez et al. (p. 533) describe the severe acute respiratory syndrome coronavirus 2 (SARS-CoV-2) infection during the first and second epidemic waves in Spain.

The REACT-1 study sampled individuals aged 5 years and older in random cross-sections of the population of England, using the National Health Service list of patients registered with a general practitioner (near-universal coverage) as a sampling frame. There were 19 rounds of data collection from May 1, 2020, to March 31, 2022. It has generated real-time data on SARS-CoV-2 prevalence over time, by area, and by sociodemographic variables; estimates of vaccine effectiveness; and symptom profiles, and it has detected emergence of new variants by viral genome sequencing.

The Spanish and British surveys are both exemplary. As stressed by Natalie Dean, Eran Bendavid, Paul Elliott, and Daniel Jernigan in related editorials (p. 514 to 523), despite specificities of the national health systems they were able to build upon, they demonstrate that it is possible to develop monitoring systems that are granular enough to track the progression of health outcomes in communities. In the absence of such population-based health monitoring, we will keep on flying blind through epidemics and pandemics. AJPH

Alfredo Morabia, MD, PhD
AJPH *Editor-in-Chief*
@AlfredoMorabia

DOI: https://doi.org/10.2105/AJPH.2023.307272

23 Years Ago

Data From State Cancer Registries

While the expanding population-based state cancer data hold great promise for cancer surveillance, various considerations influence their validity and usefulness . . . difficulties arise in coding race/ethnicity, because concepts, perceptions, methodologies, and the populations themselves change over time. . . . The method adopted in the US census is self-identification. . . . By contrast, race/ethnicity information in medical records usually represents the perception of physicians, nurses, or clerks. . . . In the case of some groups, coding is particularly susceptible to inaccuracy. For example, American Indians are frequently classified as White by health care workers. A recent report from the California Cancer Registry showed that . . . 1478 American Indian cancer cases were identified, 844 (57.1%) of which had been previously misclassified as non–American Indian cases. During its first 3 years of statewide operation, 41% (1990), 26% (1991), and 22% (1992) of reports to the North Carolina Central Cancer Registry lacked information on "Hispanic origin," which is problematic, especially in analyses of trends.

From AJPH, May 2000, p. 696

33 Years Ago

Data From Intravenous Drug Users

Intravenous drug users (IVDUs) who share injecting equipment play an important role in the transmission of [HIV-1], the causative agent of [AIDS]. There is some evidence that IVDUs are not a homogeneous group, and that sub-populations exist with different risks of infection with HIV. . . . Continued monitoring of IVDUs for HIV seroprevalence is important to identify high-risk sub-populations, to appropriately target prevention programs, and to evaluate the effectiveness of those programs. Samples of IVDUs entering drug treatment are often used for monitoring HIV exposure, partly because of their accessibility, and partly because the period before entering drug treatment is said to be characterized by a relatively high frequency of drug injection, and unsafe injection practices. . . . Use of data from drug abuse treatment programs for monitoring HIV exposure should not be adopted without further critical examination of the potential biases involved; data from drug users enrolled at different sites should not be pooled unless they have first been examined separately by site.

From AJPH, September 1990, pp. 1062 and 1066

Smallpox Immunization in Colonial America: All Too Relevant Today

Tara C. Smith, PhD

ABOUT THE AUTHOR

Tara C. Smith is with the College of Public Health, Kent State University, Kent, OH.

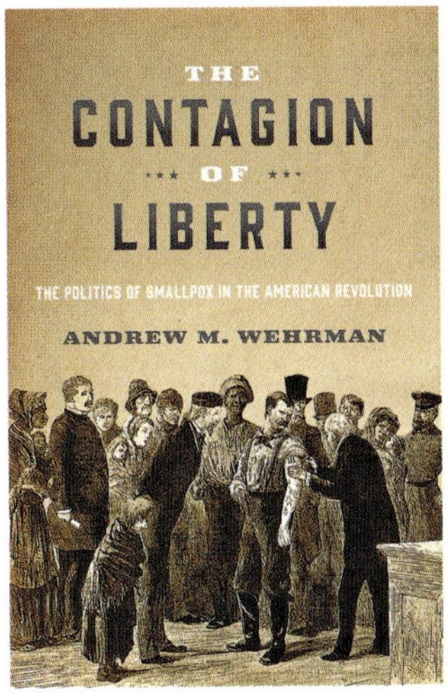

The Contagion of Liberty: The Politics of Smallpox in the American Revolution
By Andrew Wehrman
Baltimore, MD: Johns Hopkins Press; 2022
Hardcover: 401 pp; $32.00
ISBN-10: 1-4214-4466-6
ISBN-13: 978-1-4214-4466-6

Smallpox may no longer be with us, but the echoes of its effects on public health laws and vaccination campaigns remain. From colonial laws dictating rules on quarantine and isolation to 1905's *Jacobson v Massachusetts* Supreme Court case that confirmed the ability of states to mandate vaccination, the virus and response to it by government authorities and medical professionals shaped public health response in the United States.

Wehrman's thesis is that in the midst of the American Revolution, a second revolution was occurring throughout the nascent country: individuals campaigning for access to the new smallpox preventive, inoculation. Because inoculation (scratching smallpox material from an infected person into the skin) was a safer way to contract the infection, many individuals clamored for the procedure. But although inoculation was safer on an individual level, it could wreak havoc for a town, as illicit inoculation did in Boston, Massachusetts, in early 1764—potentially unleashing an outbreak, as live material was used and inoculated patients could spread the virus to others if not kept under strict isolation. Consequently, many towns, such as nearby Marblehead and Salem, Massachusetts, had strict rules to limit inoculation, generally employed when a certain threshold of families in the jurisdiction had been infected with smallpox. Boston had this restriction as well, but there were not enough people to police its larger population. For example, Paul Revere, the silversmith and patriot from Boston, was suspected of using inoculation without permission.

As Revere's (alleged) behavior demonstrates, those with means and influence could break such rules. The wealthy could afford to travel to towns where inoculation was permitted, such as areas of Pennsylvania where laws were more lax, and stay in smallpox hospitals or private residences during their convalescence that were inaccessible to those without means. The poor could neither flee nor get inoculated and were more likely to suffer from higher death rates during smallpox epidemics.

Sourced from archival documents—letters between founding fathers, newspaper articles, and more—Wehrman's book details how some of the stories about the early days of smallpox inoculation are misleading. Wehrman includes a chapter called "George Washington's About Face," describing his evolving views from skeptic of military inoculation (any soldier undergoing inoculation "must expect the severest punishment") to advocate. Washington found that inoculation was genius military strategy, and he was resigned to the fact that incoming soldiers were not going to stop inoculating. Furthermore, Washington was convinced in part because of his acquisition of a staunch proinoculation doctor as his medical advisor in late 1776, although he still wavered in January 1777 (chapter 7). Likewise, Thomas Jefferson was inoculated but believed health was a private aim rather than a public duty

AJPH May 2023, Vol 113, No. 5

and wrote nothing publicly to encourage Americans to adopt the practice.

The book shines in bringing nuance and context to these history-making decisions and demonstrates that much of the push for inoculation in the late 18th century outside the army came not from the top down via mandates but from the bottom up by vulnerable individuals clamoring for protection. Unfortunately, public health initiatives too often fizzled once the initial outcry faded, lessening in urgency after mass inoculation and even more during the early days of vaccination as yellow fever increased in incidence and miasma theory increased in popularity. Focus turned to individual diet and hygiene instead of collective action, and an attempt at a national vaccine institute designed to provide vaccination for all was underfunded and folded after just nine years.

Organized chronologically, the book is divided into 10 chapters, ranging from the introduction of inoculation in the colonies in 1721 to the replacement of inoculation with the English doctor Edward Jenner's vaccination procedure in the early 1800s. For the most part, chapters focus on a single incident or locale and a fight over inoculation and then connect that to the large picture of the smallpox revolution-within-the-revolution. Wehrman's work adds to the literature on colonial smallpox, showing how central it was to the Revolution and building on work done by Elizabeth Fenn in *Pox Americana* (2001).

Public health officials, and those with an interest in public health law in particular, would benefit from *Contagion of Liberty*. Over the past three years of the COVID-19 pandemic, controversies about preventive measures, government versus individual control of health, medical racism and health inequities, disease versus the economy, and vaccine mandates have raged. Wehrman shows that this is not new ground we are treading, although perhaps a minor flaw of the book is that connections with the COVID-19 pandemic are suggested but not explicitly discussed. Wehrman's work can help current officials understand the undercurrents of resistance and the successful (or failed) responses from centuries past and potentially inform current campaigns. AJPH

CORRESPONDENCE

Correspondence should be sent to Tara C. Smith, Lowry Hall, 750 Hilltop Dr, Kent, OH 44242 (e-mail: tsmit176@kent.edu). Reprints can be ordered at http://www.ajph.org by clicking the "Reprints" link.

PUBLICATION INFORMATION

Full Citation: Smith TC. Smallpox immunization in colonial America: all too relevant today. *Am J Public Health*. 2023;113(5):463–464.

Acceptance Date: February 16, 2023.

DOI: https://doi.org/10.2105/AJPH.2023.307264

CONFLICTS OF INTEREST

The author has no conflicts of interest to declare.

Strengthening Heat Action Plans in the United States

Melissa Guardaro, PhD, MBA

ABOUT THE AUTHOR

Melissa Guardaro is with the School of Sustainability, Arizona State University, Tempe.

See also Randazza et al., p. 559.

Extreme heat is a public health threat that extends beyond jurisdictions and institutions and has urgent short-term emergency and long-term mitigation components. Managing this issue can be problematic. Heat action plans (HAPs) are one policy tool used by public health and emergency management agencies to address the public health impacts of an increasingly warming environment. The article by Randazza et al. in this issue of *AJPH* (p. 559) examines the common content of HAPs and identifies gaps in heat preparedness.

RECOMMENDATIONS

The Centers for Disease Control and Prevention (CDC) guidance for developing HAPs details their scope and potential components, including identifying vulnerable populations, surveillance, heat-health messaging, cooling centers, and coordination among agencies.[1] Of the 21 plans analyzed by Randazza et al., the vast majority include elements recommended by the CDC and illuminate a gap between identifying vulnerable populations and outreach specifically targeted to those most at risk.

Exposure and risk levels of extreme heat are as varied as the microclimates where people reside, and solutions should reflect the local context. The effects of extreme heat are a localized issue owing to factors such as urban heat island effects, prevalence of air conditioning, energy insecurity, climate zone, development patterns, preexisting health issues, and socioeconomic factors. In the metropolitan Phoenix, Arizona, area, for example, the majority of cooling centers are open continuously from May through September, rather than being activated by National Weather Service forecasts, given the high average temperatures during that period.[2] The Maricopa County Department of Public Health reported that two thirds of heat-associated deaths occurred on days when an excessive heat warning was not issued (Figure 1).[3]

Community engagement, especially with the most heat vulnerable, should be part of the heat action planning process to ensure a local perspective in strategies deployed. Although the CDC guidance recommends targeting certain at-risk populations, its list is not exhaustive. Understanding the local setting can identify other at-risk groups. For example, in Maricopa County, mobile homes compose 4.9% of the housing stock yet account for 27.5% of the indoor heat deaths.[4] Some communities are taking action to mitigate heat in their community. Consideration should be given to community-driven HAPs that include community-vetted solutions.[5]

HEAT GOVERNANCE

The majority of the plans (81%) analyzed by Randazza et al. were led by the Office of Emergency Management, and 28% of the plans listed public health departments as having a leading role. Randazza et al. excluded plans that focused on long-term planning without addressing heat emergencies. Extreme heat is an intersectional issue. To move beyond emergency responses to extreme heat management, structural inequities and root causes need to be identified and addressed. Shifting from an emergency model to a traditional public health governance structure would promote long-term policies and help public health care systems transition to building climate change resilience.[6]

Long-term planning strategies were absent in the HAPs the authors analyzed but may be beyond the scope of emergency management or public health entities. Heat mitigation strategies, including increased use of green infrastructure, shading of public pathways, cool roofs and pavements, and energy assistance, may be better administered by municipal or regional governments. Coordination of HAPs with municipal or regional climate action plans can amplify efforts to increase thermal comfort for residents both in the short and long terms. An increasing number of municipalities are building heat response offices to coordinate actions in their city, thus breaking out of siloed decision-making to deliver more effective services.[7] Public health departments can develop

AJPH May 2023, Vol 113, No. 5

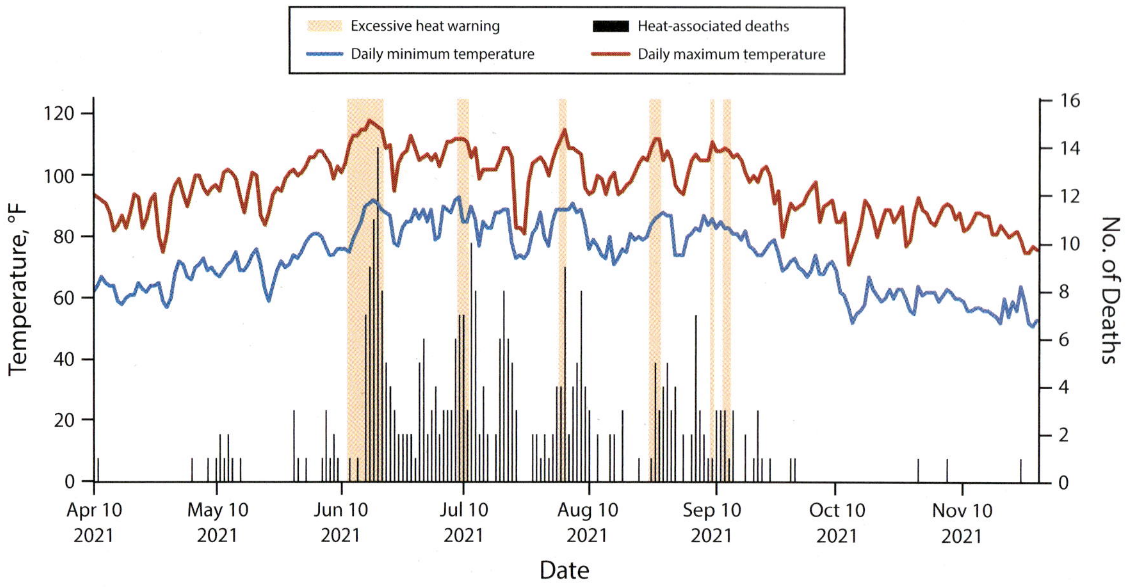

FIGURE 1— Maricopa County, Arizona, Heat-Associated Deaths and Excessive Heat Warnings: 2021

Source. Adapted from Maricopa County Public Health.[3]

similar heat response offices, which would be headed by a public health extreme heat officer with responsibility for coordinating public health heat issues.

EQUITY

Interestingly, Randazza et al. highlight the gaps between identifying at-risk populations and implementing targeting programs (see Figure 3 in Randazza et al.). This is problematic, especially because general communications can perpetuate the misunderstanding that heat warnings are not meant for these at-risk populations. The lack of heat risk perception in adults aged 65 years and older has been well documented and has been a barrier in reaching this population effectively.[8] Understanding personal risk is the first step in seeking heat-reducing programs and changing behavior.

Centering equity and environmental justice in HAPs addresses the differing heat risk between communities in the same city. Extreme heat is an equity issue that reflects historical underinvestment in infrastructure, discrimination, and lack of access to cooling amenities. HAPs can shift this dynamic by targeting historically underserved and overburdened people.[9]

SURVEILLANCE

Despite all plans calling for monitoring and surveillance, few incorporate surveillance data into the review process. HAPs compile a range of data from National Weather Service forecasts, heat-health data such as heat-related emergency department visits, monitoring of at-risk populations such as those experiencing homelessness, and information on cooling center use, utility infrastructure, and police and fire department calls. Along with these measures for managing heat as an emergency situation, other data should be part of the decision-making process to gauge changing demographics, institutional capabilities, funding, and increased incidences of hazards, which could guide a coordinated, collaborative, comprehensive extreme heat response.

CONCLUSIONS

HAPs present an opportunity to address the growing public health crisis. Caution should be taken when developing the HAPs to go beyond business as usual to reflect the needs and context of local communities. HAPs should be examined holistically to measure the effect of a coordinated response and synergies with other heat policy tools, such as climate action plans. Given climate predictions, the HAPs are one important path to improving public health outcomes and increasing climate resilience. AJPH

CORRESPONDENCE

Correspondence should be sent to Melissa Guardaro, School of Sustainability, Arizona State University, Walton Center for Planetary Health, 777 E. University Dr, Tempe, AZ 85281 (e-mail: melissa.guardaro@asu.edu). Reprints can be ordered at http://www.ajph.org by clicking the "Reprints" link.

PUBLICATION INFORMATION

Full Citation: Guardaro M. Strengthening heat action plans in the United States. *Am J Public Health*. 2023;113(5):465–467.

Acceptance Date: February 12, 2023.

DOI: https://doi.org/10.2105/AJPH.2023.307260

ACKNOWLEDGMENTS

I would like to recognize the collaborative work of the Arizona Heat Resilience Working Group and the Arizona Cooling Center Working Group.

CONFLICTS OF INTEREST

The author has no conflicts of interest to disclose.

REFERENCES

1. Abbinett J, Schramm PJ, Widerynski S. Heat response plans: summary of evidence and strategies for collaboration and implementation. 2020. Available at: https://www.cdc.gov/climateandhealth/docs/HeatResponsePlans_508.pdf. Accessed February 22, 2023.
2. Maricopa Association of Governments. Heat Relief Network. Available at: https://hrn.azmag.gov. Accessed February 22, 2023.
3. Maricopa County Department of Public Health. Heat-associated deaths in Maricopa County, AZ. Final Report for 2021. Available at: https://www.maricopa.gov/ArchiveCenter/ViewFile/Item/5494. Accessed February 22, 2023.
4. Phillips LA, Solís P, Wang C, Varfalameyeva K, Burnett J. Engaged convergence research: an exploratory approach to heat resilience in mobile homes. *Prof Geogr*. 2021;73(4):619–631. https://doi.org/10.1080/00330124.2021.1924805
5. Guardaro M, Messerschmidt M, Hondula DM, Grimm NB, Redman CL. Building community heat action plans story by story: a three neighborhood case study. *Cities*. 2020;107:102886. https://doi.org/10.1016/j.cities.2020.102886
6. Schmeltz MT, Smith JA, Olmos I, Quintero E. Extreme heat governance: a critical analysis of heat action plans in California. *Am J Public Health*. 2023;113(1):15–19. https://doi.org/10.2105/AJPH.2022.307117
7. Keith L, Meerow S, Hondula DM, Turner VK, Arnott JC. Deploy heat officers, policies and metrics. *Nature*. 2021;598(7879):29–31. https://doi.org/10.1038/d41586-021-02677-2
8. Howe PD, Marlon JR, Wang X, Leiserowitz A. Public perceptions of the health risks of extreme heat across US states, counties, and neighborhoods. *Proc Natl Acad Sci U S A*. 2019;116(14):6743–6748. https://doi.org/10.1073/pnas.1813145116
9. US Environmental Protection Agency. Heat islands and equity. December 12. 2022. Available at: https://www.epa.gov/heatislands/heat-islands-and-equity. Accessed February 22, 2023.

Translating Hannah Stone's Patient-Centric Values to the Widest Possible Audience of Young People—In the Classroom as Well as the Clinic

Ellen S. More, PhD

ABOUT THE AUTHOR

The author is professor emeritus, University of Massachusetts Chan Medical School, Worcester.

AJPH May 2023, Vol 113, No. 5

"I knew about birth control because I had been to see the great Hannah Stone as a patient." Those words could have been spoken by any one of thousands of New York City women between 1925 and 1941. As it happened, they were spoken by Mary Steichen Calderone, first medical director of the Planned Parenthood Federation of America (1953–1964) and cofounder in 1964 of the Sexuality Information and Education Council of the United States (SIECUS). Calderone added, "[Hannah Stone] fitted me with a diaphragm, of course."[1]

As Robin E. Jensen describes in "The First Publication on Contraception in a US Medical Journal, 1928: Hannah Mayer Stone's Case for Contraceptive Care Before the Pill,"[2] Hannah Stone was one of the great pioneers of contraceptive medicine in the 20th century. Today, in the wake of the US Supreme Court's 2022 *Dobbs* decision, when access to reproductive health care cannot be taken for granted, Stone's example takes on renewed importance.

Her contributions were often overshadowed by figures such as Margaret Sanger, for whom she worked at the Clinical Research Bureau of the American Birth Control League in New York City, and Robert Latou Dickinson, MD, an advocate for birth control as part of good medical practice and founder of the Committee on Maternal Health. Yet, at great legal and professional risk, Stone laid the groundwork for medically sound contraceptive care. Her 1928 article was the first published account demonstrating the effectiveness and safety of contraceptive methods antecedent to the birth control pill in 1960. Just as important, her work was a model for individualized, patient-centered care.

Disregarding the risks to her career—not only was Stone one of a minority of women among practitioners in the United States in the interwar years (4.4% in 1930),[3] she chose to work in the professional hinterlands of contraceptive medicine—Stone made a signal contribution to the eventual acceptance of birth control as part of public health and private practice. She created a network of likeminded practitioners who would, she hoped, replicate her findings and expand the availability of effective birth control.

At the heart of Stone's success was a steadfast commitment to careful recordkeeping and follow-up with her patients, a precursor to clinical research. She and her husband, Abraham Stone, MD, published a highly regarded sex-and-marriage manual based on counseling many hundreds of couples.[4] In her birth control practice, too, Stone listened to her patients and modified her practices in response to their feedback. Her patients rewarded her care with high rates of adherence, providing her with the data to make a "pioneer contribution," in Dickinson's words, to the published literature on contraception.[5]

Stone's achievements were significant but preliminary. Widespread recognition of birth control as a part of good medical practice became evident after 1959 when the American Public Health Association endorsed it. The American Medical Association followed suit in 1964 (two years after the pill became available), but only after joint efforts by Calderone, Janet Dingle, and others to persuade its leaders to amend the organization's policy.[6]

As Jensen writes, Stone worked from the principle that "effective provision of contraceptive care always starts and stops with attention to the experiences and needs of individual patients."[7(p. 395)] Subsequent generations of birth control advocates, however, have learned another lesson: that contraceptive health care, indeed sexual health care more generally, begins long before anyone becomes a "patient."

According to a recent survey, three quarters of American youths 13 to 17 years of age have accessed pornography online.[8] At least up to the onset of the COVID-19 pandemic, more than half of the students in that age group participated in sexual activity in some form.[9] Preserving their sexual health requires engaging with students about facts and values related to sexuality; the conversation must begin long before they visit a doctor's office or a clinic. They need access to scientifically sound, age-appropriate, gender-inclusive, and comprehensive sex education. They are more likely to receive it—if they do—in schools than in their homes or religious institutions.[10]

Sex education has been at the heart of some of the most divisive battles in American school systems, particularly since the early 1960s. Sex education advocates such as SIECUS have attempted to balance a focus on basic anatomy lessons, pregnancy prevention, and reductions in sexually transmitted infections with topics such as healthy attitudes, self-esteem, and communication skills. That has been a mostly losing battle, and not just because of the successes of social conservatives in establishing "abstinence-only" and "abstinence-plus" curricula. Americans are simply uncomfortable talking about sexuality as what Calderone called a "health entity."

The origins of "comprehensive" sex education track closely with the growing concern over safe sexual practices in response to the dangers of HIV/AIDS.[11] Since 1989, architects of sex education have focused on curricular goals that could be measured and compared with abstinence-only sex education, especially a curriculum's effectiveness in delaying the onset of sexual activity, unwanted pregnancies, and sexually transmitted infections.[12] In today's world, demands for reproductive justice cannot be met unless all students can access reliable information that enables them to achieve the goal of sexual health in an atmosphere that conveys information without evoking shame or fear of sexuality. Stone helped begin this process, patient by patient. Today we need to translate her patient-centric values to the widest possible audience of young people in both the classroom and the clinic. AJPH

CORRESPONDENCE

Correspondence should be sent to Ellen S. More, PhD, 521 Salisbury St, Worcester, MA 01609 (e-mail: ellen.more@umassmed.edu). Reprints can be ordered at http://www.ajph.org by clicking the "Reprints" link.

PUBLICATION INFORMATION

Full Citation: More ES. Translating Hannah Stone's patient-centric values to the widest possible audience of young people—in the classroom as well as the clinic. *Am J Public Health*. 2023;113(5): 468–469.

Acceptance Date: January 29, 2023.

DOI: https://doi.org/10.2105/AJPH.2023.307248

CONFLICTS OF INTEREST

The author has no conflicts of interest to declare.

ENDNOTES

1. "Mary Steichen Calderone," in Lynn Gilbert and Gaylen Moore, eds., *Particular Passions: Talks with Women Who Have Shaped Our Times* (New York, NY: Clarkson N. Potter, 1982), 255–263, quotation 257.
2. Robin E. Jensen, "The First Publication on Contraception in a US Medical Journal, 1928: Hannah Mayer Stone's Case for Contraceptive Care Before the Pill," *Am J Public Health*. 2023;113(4): 390–396.
3. Ellen S. More, Elizabeth Fee, and Manon Parry, "Introduction," in Ellen S. More, Elizabeth Fee, and Manon Parry, eds., *Women Physicians and the Cultures of Medicine* (Baltimore, MD: Johns Hopkins University Press, 2009), 1–20, Table 1.1.
4. Hannah M. Stone and Abraham Stone, *A Marriage Manual: A Guide-Book to Sex and Marriage*, rev. ed. (New York, NY: Simon and Schuster, 1939).
5. Robert L. Dickinson, "Open Forum: Birth Control," *Medical Journal and Record* (March 1928): 9.
6. Ellen S. More, *The Transformation of American Sex Education: Mary Calderone and the Fight for Sexual Health* (New York, NY: New York University, 2022), 42–47, 69, 70. At the time, Calderone was the medical director of the Planned Parenthood Federation of America and Dingle headed the federation's Cleveland affiliate.
7. Jensen, "The First Publication on Contraception in a US Medical Journal," 395.
8. Cecilia Kang, "Most Teenagers Have Seen Online Porn, Report Says," *New York Times*, January 10, 2023, B1, B4.
9. Laura D. Lindberg, Lauren Firestine, and Cynthia Beavin, "Trends in US Adolescent Sexual Behavior and Contraceptive Use, 2009–2019" (https://www.sciencedirect.com/science/article/pii/S2590151621000113), accessed January 21, 2023. Adolescent sexual activity has been reported to have declined during the pandemic.
10. More, *The Transformation of American Sex Education*.
11. More, *The Transformation of American Sex Education*, 217–218.
12. Douglas Kirby, *Emerging Answers 2007: Research Findings on Programs to Reduce Teen Pregnancy and Sexually Transmitted Disease* (Washington, DC: National Campaign to Prevent Teen and Unplanned Pregnancy, 2007); Eva S. Goldfarb and Lisa D. Lieberman, "Three Decades of Research: The Case for Comprehensive Sex Education," *Journal of Adolescent Health* 68 (2021): 13–27.

Centering Patients' Voices in Artificial Intelligence–Based Telemedicine

Stephanie A. Kraft, JD

ABOUT THE AUTHOR

Stephanie A. Kraft is with the Treuman Katz Center for Pediatric Bioethics, Seattle Children's Research Institute, and the Department of Pediatrics, School of Medicine, University of Washington, Seattle.

See also Tiribelli et al., p. 577.

Artificial intelligence (AI) and telemedicine, individually and together, are rapidly changing how patients interact with the health care system. AI coupled with health care delivery via telemedicine can help promote shared decision-making by bringing data-informed predictions to patients and their providers.[1] These technologies have potential to improve meaningful access to quality care by meeting patients where they are and empowering them, in collaboration with their providers, to take steps toward promoting their health.

Yet AI-powered health care also has potential to exacerbate existing health care disparities,[2] cause harm to patients, and fail to serve the health of the public if it is not designed and deployed with attention to patients' values, needs, and priorities. In doing so, these technologies may not only cause harm but also may undermine public trust in AI in medicine. The recent proliferation of AI-powered chatbots illustrates the simultaneous power of AI and its potential threats to trust in science and medicine. The journal *Nature*, for example, recently issued guidance for transparency around the use of chatbots in producing scientific work out of a recognition that their use could signal a lack of scientific integrity and trustworthiness.[3]

AI in health care delivery similarly has great potential to support clinical communication and decision-making, but it is easy to imagine how its use could convey insincerity, provide inaccurate or unhelpful information, or otherwise undermine a therapeutic patient–provider relationship. Indeed, trustworthy AI in medicine requires attention not just to considerations such as transparency of the AI itself but also to how its use affects patients' experiences receiving care, their ability to make autonomous decisions, and health equity across society more broadly. Trustworthy medical AI must incorporate a nuanced understanding of people's health care experiences—which previous qualitative work has shown can be influenced by multiple factors at both the interpersonal and organizational levels[4]—and how AI may change them. A holistic approach that recognizes the interplay among technology, policy, and interpersonal relationships is essential to understand how AI affects patients' experiences and ability to trust in the care they are receiving.

BEGINNING WITH RELIABILITY AND RELATIONSHIPS

Centering the conversation around trust, however, may not be enough. As Kerasidou et al.[5] argue, focusing on trust overlooks a critical systems-level responsibility: reliability. That is, before we can begin talking about earning patients' trust, AI in health care must be scaffolded by robust regulatory and ethical oversight and accountability. In their article, Tiribelli et al. (p. 577) offer an ethical framework for how to work toward such reliability for AI-based telemedicine, a context in which there has previously been little attention paid to understanding the nuances of how to ethically deploy AI. Telemedicine is a key patient-facing technology—made even more important throughout the COVID-19 pandemic—in which the technology mediates patients' interactions with their health care providers, alleviating some barriers to health care while in some cases introducing others. Recognizing that reliability is essential for AI-based telemedicine, and yet existing ethical frameworks have not been tailored to its unique considerations, Tiribelli et al. synthesize frameworks from multiple disciplines to examine what reliable ethical oversight should look like in this setting.

In discussing their framework, the authors note the importance of recognizing patients' social situatedness and using a relational autonomy lens to understand how people make health care decisions. Even beyond autonomous decision-making, relational ethics can offer a broader appreciation of how to

AJPH May 2023, Vol 113, No. 5

develop ethical guidelines that will maximize benefits and minimize harms that are most impactful for patients. A relational lens reminds us that patients, providers, technology developers, regulators, and indeed all of us are informed by the social context in which we live and our relationships with one another.[6] Technology is not values-neutral; rather, it reflects the values of those who create it, those who collected the data that it builds on, and the sociopolitical context for which it is tailored. In their article, Tiribelli et al. offer an approach to break down some of the values embedded within AI-based telemedicine and illustrate that it raises perpetual ethical questions of what the impact of medical technology is on patients and how it ought to be designed and implemented to promote ethical and equitable health care.

INTEGRATING DIVERSE PATIENT VOICES

Key to addressing these questions is the voice of the patient—or rather, many voices of many patients. If medical technology is meant to help patients flourish, it needs to recognize and make space for the diversity of ways in which people flourish, as well as the things that prevent people from flourishing. Societal systems of oppression including, but not limited to, racism, sexism, and ableism have well-documented impacts on people's health as well as their ability to engage safely and effectively with the health care system; a robust appreciation of these systems and their impacts is necessary if AI-based telemedicine is to work toward dismantling them and advancing health equity.[7]

In applying their framework, Tiribelli et al. rightly highlight the importance of "equity in user representation with specific attention to the inclusion of marginalized/vulnerable groups" during the process of technology design and deployment. This work of understanding patients' lived experiences must be foundational to the development of medical technology and particularly AI-based technologies that have potential to amplify and further embed existing disparities. This will require a commitment to patient- and community-engaged research on the part of those who develop, implement, and fund medical AI. This work need not start from scratch, but can build on the groundwork, missteps, and lessons learned in fields like genetics, which has navigated ethical questions about accuracy, utility, and social implications of predictive testing for more than 30 years. Key among these lessons is that it is critical to engage with a diverse range of patients and communities, especially those who have been marginalized and mistreated in medicine, early and often throughout the development process to identify priorities, ensure usability, and minimize harms.

Health care systems have long failed their most marginalized patients, and new technology gives us the opportunity—and obligation—to do better. Building AI with patient voices at the center is essential to ensure it neither contributes to nor is indifferent to the failures of the past and present, but instead is working to advance inclusivity and justice in health care. As we continue to learn about the impacts of AI on patients and their communities, and as technology and health care systems evolve, ethical frameworks that allow us to be responsive to these changing needs will be best situated to promote reliability and support medical AI that, over time, can show itself to be worthy of patients' trust. AJPH

CORRESPONDENCE

Correspondence should be sent to Stephanie A. Kraft, c/o Seattle Children's Research Institute, 1900 Ninth Ave, M/S JMB-6, Seattle, WA 98101 (e-mail: stephanie.kraft@seattlechildrens.org). Reprints can be ordered at https://ajph.org by clicking the "Reprints" link.

PUBLICATION INFORMATION

Full Citation: Kraft SA. Centering patients' voices in artificial intelligence–based telemedicine. *Am J Public Health*. 2023;113(5):470–471.

Acceptance Date: February 16, 2023.

DOI: https://doi.org/10.2105/AJPH.2023.307270

ACKNOWLEDGMENTS

Thank you to the editorial team for their invitation to write this piece and to my many collaborators and colleagues whose discussions over the years have helped these ideas develop.

CONFLICTS OF INTEREST

There are no conflicts of interest related to this work.

REFERENCES

1. Abbasgholizadeh Rahimi S, Cwintal M, Huang Y, et al. Application of artificial intelligence in shared decision making: scoping review. *JMIR Med Inform*. 2022;10(8):e36199. https://doi.org/10.2196/36199
2. Obermeyer Z, Powers B, Vogeli C, Mullainathan S. Dissecting racial bias in an algorithm used to manage the health of populations. *Science*. 2019; 366(6464):447–453. https://doi.org/10.1126/science.aax2342
3. Tools such as ChatGPT threaten transparent science; here are our ground rules for their use. *Nature*. 2023;613(7945):61. https://doi.org/10.1038/d41586-023-00191-1
4. Bridges C, Duenas DM, Lewis H, et al. Patient perspectives on how to demonstrate respect: implications for clinicians and healthcare organizations. *PLoS One*. 2021;16(4):e0250999. https://doi.org/10.1371/journal.pone.0250999
5. Kerasidou CX, Kerasidou A, Buscher M, Wilkinson S. Before and beyond trust: reliance in medical AI. *J Med Ethics*. 2022;48(11):852–856. https://doi.org/10.1136/medethics-2020-107095
6. Campelia GD, Feinsinger A. Creating space for feminist ethics in medical school. *HEC Forum*. 2020;32(2):111–124. https://doi.org/10.1007/s10730-020-09403-x
7. Figueroa CA, Luo T, Aguilera A, Lyles CR. The need for feminist intersectionality in digital health. *Lancet Digit Health*. 2021;3(8):e526–e533. https://doi.org/10.1016/S2589-7500(21)00118-7

To End Youth Vaping as an On-Ramp to Addiction, Close Legal Loopholes and Rigorously Enforce the Law

Mark A. Gottlieb, JD

ABOUT THE AUTHOR

Mark A. Gottlieb is with the Public Health Advocacy Institute, Northeastern University School of Law, Boston, MA.

See also Azagba et al., p. 568.

AJPH May 2023, Vol 113, No. 5

The business of selling flavored e-cigarettes to youths is built on a foundation of loopholes. In this issue, Azagba et al. (p. 568) discuss their thorough review of state laws and legal loopholes in the final step of the distribution chain that begins with e-cigarette manufacture and ends with delivery to vaping adolescents. This public health problem was avoidable, but because of a combination of gaps, loopholes, and uneven enforcement, millions of young people are now nicotine dependent despite never smoking a cigarette.

The legal landscape of e-cigarettes in the United States has been in disarray ever since the introduction of the product to the market in early 2007. At that time, there were no state laws addressing the sale or use of these novel nicotine delivery devices. In 2008, the US Food and Drug Administration (FDA) sought to halt e-cigarette importation as a drug delivery device without approval and, in response, manufacturers filed a legal challenge to the FDA. While that lawsuit was pending, Congress passed the Smoking Prevention and Tobacco Control Act of 2009, which granted the FDA regulatory authority over tobacco products. In 2010, an appeals court ruled that the FDA should regulate e-cigarettes as tobacco products rather than drug delivery devices.[1]

Under the act, to regulate anything other than cigarettes or smokeless tobacco, the FDA first must engage in a rule-making process to deem them to be tobacco products. This took the agency six years to complete while e-cigarette sales grew sevenfold.[2] During this time, devices rapidly evolved into sleek, flavored, and palatable high-dose rapid nicotine delivery systems that youths found socially and physiologically compelling.[3] Juul introduced its product to the market in 2015 with more than twice the nicotine concentration of its competitors and quickly gained 75% of the US e-cigarette market.[4] By 2018, the US Surgeon General characterized youth vaping as an epidemic.[5]

The overwhelming majority of vaping adolescents were using e-cigarette products with flavors such as fruit, mango, and mint.[6] The FDA announced in early 2020 that it would no longer permit pod-based e-cigarette producers such as Juul to sell their products with flavors other than tobacco or menthol varieties.[7] For reasons not well understood, the FDA exempted single-use flavored e-cigarette products known as "disposables" from its enforcement plan. Because of this loophole, high school students' use of flavored disposables quickly increased 10-fold in 2020.[8] Puff Bar, a leading disposable brand that sold all of the prohibited Juul flavors and more, became the top-selling e-cigarette brand among youths.[8] Shortly thereafter, the FDA issued warning letters to Puff Bar and other sellers of disposable flavored e-cigarettes because, as it turns out, none of those products were authorized for sale by the FDA or otherwise eligible to be legally sold.[9] Puff Bar quickly discontinued online sales. This closed a gaping loophole. Or did it?

In 2021, Puff Bar and other disposable flavored e-cigarette makers found another loophole to exploit and quickly returned to the market with products they claimed used nicotine that was not derived from tobacco, which, they argued, exempted them from the FDA's regulatory authority over tobacco products.[10] These flavored e-cigarettes were available both at retail and a seemingly endless number of online vendors. Congress, as part of the Consolidated Appropriations Act of 2022, sought to close this loophole by granting the FDA explicit regulatory authority over nicotine-containing tobacco products regardless of the nicotine's source. Although this law went into effect in April 2022, flavored disposable e-cigarettes continue to be readily available online and in stores. The FDA states that it received approximately one million applications for nontobacco nicotine in 2022, and, as of February 2023, none has received marketing authorizations from the agency.[11] Although it appears that these federal legal loopholes permitting sales of flavored e-cigarettes have been closed, a significant and persistent enforcement operation is needed to stop unauthorized product sales.

Although it is not legal to sell tobacco products to persons younger than 21 years, adolescents still get them, often through online sales.[12] At the federal level, Congress passed a law in 2020, the Preventing Online Sales of E-Cigarettes to Children Act, which resulted in the US Postal Service and major parcel delivery companies excluding themselves from e-cigarette delivery operations. But, as Azagba et al. note, independently contracted drivers have found a regulatory gap to continue e-cigarette deliveries from online and telephone purchases. This gap theoretically can be closed at the state level, and the authors found that, indeed, 34 states have passed such laws, with 27 of them requiring age verification for delivery, a critical provision to include.

Azagba et al. observe that inconsistencies in state law provisions leave unfortunate loopholes or, where enforcement of the law is lacking, the potential to simply disregard such laws. This points to a need for model legislation to be established and widely adopted to close loopholes and provide strong but practical enforcement procedures and penalties. Although enormous challenges remain upstream as the FDA seeks to get a handle on controlling unauthorized sales of flavored e-cigarettes, the work of Azagba et al. reminds us that there are concrete steps that can be taken at the state level to reduce the volume of e-cigarettes reaching youths. In addition to delivery laws, comprehensive flavor bans such as those enacted in California and Massachusetts provide a way to reduce access to the products that are most responsible for youth initiation and dependence on tobacco products. *AJPH*

CORRESPONDENCE

Correspondence should be sent to Mark A. Gottlieb, Public Health Advocacy Institute at Northeastern University School of Law, 360 Huntington Ave, Suite 117CU, Boston MA 02115-5005 (e-mail: ma.gottlieb@northeastern.edu). Reprints can be ordered at http://www.ajph.org by clicking the "Reprints" link.

PUBLICATION INFORMATION

Full Citation: Gottlieb MA. To end youth vaping as an on-ramp to addiction, close legal loopholes and rigorously enforce the law. *Am J Public Health*. 2023;113(5):472–473.

Acceptance Date: February 16, 2023.

DOI: https://doi.org/10.2105/AJPH.2023.307271

ACKNOWLEDGMENTS

The author wishes to express gratitude to his long-time colleague, Richard A. Daynard, for his many years of encouragement and inspiration.

CONFLICTS OF INTEREST

The author has no conflicts of interest to report.

REFERENCES

1. *Sottera, Inc. v US Food and Drug Administration*. 627 F.3d 891 (D.C. Cir, 2010). Available at: https://www.courtlistener.com/opinion/180504/sottera-inc-v-food-drug-admin. Accessed January 28, 2023.
2. Cantrell J, Huang J, Greenberg M, Willett J, Hair E, Vallone D. History and current trends in the electronic cigarette retail marketplace in the United States: 2010–2016. *Nicotine Tob Res*. 2020;22(5):843–847. https://doi.org/10.1093/ntr/nty214
3. Malek N, Nakkash R, Talih S, et al. A transdisciplinary approach to understanding characteristics of electronic cigarettes. *Tob Regul Sci*. 2018;4(3):47–72. https://doi.org/10.18001/TRS.4.3.5
4. Jackler RK, Ramamurthi D. Nicotine arms race: JUUL and the high-nicotine product market. *Tob Control*. 2019;28(6):623–628. https://doi.org/10.1136/tobaccocontrol-2018-054796
5. US Surgeon General. Surgeon general's advisory on e-cigarette use among youth. 2018. Available at: https://e-cigarettes.surgeongeneral.gov/documents/surgeon-generals-advisory-on-e-cigarette-use-among-youth-2018.pdf. Accessed January 19, 2023.
6. Cullen KA, Gentzke AS, Sawdey MD, et al. E-Cigarette use among youth in the United States, 2019. *JAMA*. 2019;322(21):2095. https://doi.org/10.1001/jama.2019.18387
7. US Food and Drug Administration. Enforcement priorities for electronic nicotine delivery system (ENDS) and other deemed products on the market without premarket authorization. April 2020. Available at: https://www.fda.gov/regulatory-information/search-fda-guidance-documents/enforcement-priorities-electronic-nicotine-delivery-system-ends-and-other-deemed-products-market. Accessed January 30, 2023.
8. Centers for Disease Control and Prevention. Notes from the field: e-cigarette use among middle and high school students—National Youth Tobacco Survey, United States, 2021. *MMWR Morb Mortal Wkly Rep*. 2021;70(39):1387–1389. https://doi.org/10.15585/mmwr.mm7039a4
9. US Food and Drug Administration. Warning letter to Cool Clouds Distribution, Inc. d/b/a Puff Bar. MARCS-CMS 608526. July 20, 2020. Available at: https://www.fda.gov/inspections-compliance-enforcement-and-criminal-investigations/warning-letters/cool-clouds-distribution-inc-dba-puff-bar-608526-07202020. Accessed February 2, 2023.
10. Kong G, Krishnan-Sarin S. Tobacco free nicotine (TFN): a new public health challenge. July 3, 2021. Available at: https://blogs.bmj.com/tc/2021/07/03/tobacco-free-nicotine-tfn-a-new-public-health-challenge. Accessed January 30, 2023.
11. US Food and Drug Administration. Regulation and enforcement of non-tobacco nicotine (NTN) products. Available at: https://www.fda.gov/tobacco-products/products-ingredients-components/regulation-and-enforcement-non-tobacco-nicotine-ntn-products. Accessed February 3, 2023.
12. Gaiha SM, Henriksen L, Halpern-Felsher B, et al. Sources of flavoured e-cigarettes among California youth and young adults: associations with local flavoured tobacco sales restrictions. *Tob Control*. 2022;31(5):659–662. https://doi.org/10.1136/tobaccocontrol-2020-056455

Looking Back: Intimate Partner Violence in Transgender Populations

B. Ethan Coston, PhD

ABOUT THE AUTHOR

B. Ethan Coston is with the Department of Gender, Sexuality and Women's Studies, Virginia Commonwealth University, Richmond.

In 2020, Peitzmeier et al.[1] published a systematic review and meta-analysis of the prevalence and correlates of intimate partner violence (IPV) against transgender people. Their article garnered wide public engagement, and Altmetric currently scores it as in the top 5% of all research outputs. It was groundbreaking in its methodological approach, presenting data that were "publicly available for the first time from more than 40% of included studies and leverag[ing] data from almost 50 000 transgender respondents."[1(pe11)]

Among the various central findings, the authors report that transgender individuals are more than twice as likely as cisgender individuals to experience physical and sexual IPV in their lifetimes. For school-based samples (middle school, high school, and college), they found that transgender students and youths were up to 3.9 times more likely to experience IPV than were their cisgender peers.

I provide some context for why these findings have been so widely cited and shared, and for how the article remains relevant to explaining some of the sources of today's continued attacks on transgender people and transgender rights.

THIS MOMENT IN TRANSGENDER HISTORY

Although we would not have used the same terms, and the individuals themselves would not have understood gender the way we do today (because gender itself is always culturally and historically situated), we can definitively say that transgender people have always existed.[2–6] So why, then, are transgender people only recently increasingly the focus of politicians' campaigns, parents' self-help Facebook groups, pop cultures' commentary, gun-toting extremists' protests, and legislator's public agendas?

The answer lies, in part, in what some describe as the backlash theory of politics, or

> a particular form of political contestation with a retrograde objective as well as extraordinary goals or tactics that has reached the threshold level of entering mainstream public discourse.[7(p740)]

We are seeing that as more transgender people—particularly youths—announce their presence to the world, attempt to claim positions of political power, and are represented in popular culture (e.g., on TV shows, in fashion), those who are fearful of gender fluidity or ignorant about gender itself make arguments for a return to "simpler" or "more Christian" times. Embedded in these arguments is the belief that transgender people are harmful, lying, deceitful, predatory (e.g., not Christian) others and that transness itself is a contagion to be culled.[8] These arguments harken to a time (retrograde) when transgender people certainly existed but were largely and often purposely hidden from social view. In reality, transgender people were violently forced to be "deceitful" to obtain care, and, in the process, have been erased from history.[9]

Still, this rhetoric has terrifying carceral–legal impacts. Each year since the 2020 presidential election, when a vehemently antitransgender president lost reelection, the United States has seen a record-breaking number of antitransgender laws, bills, and executive orders introduced.[9,10] For a while, antitransgender legislation remained fairly stable, approximately 20 bills each year from 2015 to 2019.[9,11] Then there were 60 in 2020, 131 in 2021, 183 in 2022, and 371 in the first two months of 2023.[9] Although many of the bills have been dead on arrival, we have seen the passage of legislation in 23 states across the United States that restricts transgender youths' access to equitable education and extracurricular sports activities, prevents transgender adults from changing their identification documents and being able to adopt children, and criminalizes the health care workers and facilities that provide gender-affirming care.[9]

SCORNED LOVERS AND INTIMATE OTHERS

The belief that we are deceitful, violent, and predatory, supported by legal intervention, permeates every aspect of the interpersonal, familial, and communal spheres. For 21 years, the National Coalition of Anti-Violence Programs found that bias-motivated murders against transgender people, particularly transgender women of color, were increasing. In their most recent report, more than half of all murders occurred at the hands of a known offender or dating partner (including first meetups).[12] For hate violence that did not result in murder, 20% were committed by family members or relatives, 13% were committed by a friend, and 12% were committed by a current or former lover or partner.[11] For violence reported as intimate and from a partner (i.e., not reported as a hate violence incident), 33% involved antitransgender bias in the offender's tactics.[11]

For transgender people, hate violence is often intimate, and intimate violence is often imbued with hate. The piece by Peitzmeier et al. confirms this, finding that IPV victimization was associated with bullying, family assault, family harassment, general violence victimization, repeated gender-related victimization, and everyday discrimination. There have been a handful of prominent headlines throughout the years that bolster the claim that intimate partner and hate violence are bound up with one another. The *Washington Post* also recently found that nearly half of all transgender women killed between 2015 and 2020 died at the hands of an intimate partner.[13]

Scorned exes and former intimate partners of transgender people commit all kinds of violence in the aftermath of relationships, not just murder. One of the most famous examples of such a scorned ex is said to be Janice Raymond. In 1979, Raymond—a 35-year-old self-identified radical lesbian feminist and assistant professor of women's studies at the University of Massachusetts, Amherst—published a book based on her dissertation, titled *The Transsexual Empire: The Making of the She-Male*. In it, she argued that the existence of transgender people (largely she writes only about transgender women) reinforces the patriarchal oppression of (cisgender—although she does not use this word) women and constitutes a symbolic act of sexual violence against them.

The Transsexual Empire thrust Raymond into the political milieu, and in 1980 she was asked to write a report for the National Center for Health Care Technology that was funded by the US government. In this report, which was titled "Technology on the Social and Ethical Aspects of Transsexual Surgery," she argued that medical intervention for transsexual people is an ethical issue that raises "questions of bodily mutilation," and she ultimately called for "the elimination of transsexualism."[14] Her report and conclusions were used as the foundation for Medicare's blanket exclusion of transgender health care coverage—which was not lifted until 2016.

Why is this story about Raymond important? Julia Serano recently wrote a Twitter thread about how she discovered, when doing research for her own book *Whipping Girl* (2007), numerous references that suggested Raymond had either "been dumped by a trans woman she was dating" or had been left by her "cis female partner" "for a trans woman" before finishing and publishing *The Transsexual Empire*. It would seem that personal experiences with transgender people are what fanned the public, social, and political flames of Raymond's antitransgender bias.

Unfortunately, as Peitzmeier et al. found, there is little work being done to identify and better understand the characteristics, motivations, biases, beliefs, cognitive processes of abusive partners and the potential opportunities to prevent or intervene in their violence. In fact, "no studies included in the review explored the characteristics of abusive partners for transgender victims of IPV," and no study has "developed or tested the efficacy of transgender-specific IPV primary prevention interventions."[1(pe10)]

QUELLING TRANSGENDER ANTAGONISM

Transgender antagonism is everywhere today.[15] This is also an important aspect of the findings of Peitzmeier et al.: those who experience IPV are often left isolated and without care in the aftermath. Discrimination in IPV and domestic violence shelters is common, especially for transgender women, those perceived by others as transgender, disabled individuals, and indigenous, multiracial, and Latine survivors. Service providers, ranging from shelter staff to law enforcement officials, report feeling uncomfortable serving transgender clients, and nurses trained specifically in sexual assault forensics report being unprepared to work with transgender patients. With the known risks of engaging with the police, and histories of familial rejection, transgender people may have nowhere to turn when faced with a violent partner.

This lack of knowledge, training, and willingness to effectively serve transgender survivors has wide-reaching effects. The studies analyzed by Peitzmeier et al. show that experiencing IPV, in the confines of this transgender antagonism, increases the risk of reporting poorer physical, sexual, and mental health outcomes as well as being more likely to report using substances to cope. Given this, they conclude:

> Efforts are needed to develop transgender-specific, transgender-inclusive, and transgender-led interventions for IPV prevention, screening, reporting, and response in transgender populations worldwide.[1(pe11)]

COMMUNITY INVOLVEMENT AND CHANGE

A key takeaway from the work of Peitzmeier et al. is that we (all) must end the epidemic of antitransgender violence and that we (transgender people) cannot do it alone. It is far past time for every scholar, activist, service provider, health care worker, politician, and community member to come together to address this critical public health and human rights concern.

For additional resources, informational guides and reports, organizations, and service providers, and to learn how to get involved nationally or in your local area, start by visiting the National Sexual Violence Resource Center's transgender survivor support page.[16] AJPH

CORRESPONDENCE

Correspondence should be sent to B. Ethan Coston, Box 843060, Richmond, VA 23284-3060 (e-mail: bmcoston@vcu.edu). Reprints can be ordered at http://www.ajph.org by clicking the "Reprints" link.

PUBLICATION INFORMATION

Full Citation: BE Coston. Looking back: intimate partner violence in transgender populations. *Am J Public Health.* 2023;113(5):474–476.

Acceptance Date: February 14, 2023.

DOI: https://doi.org/10.2105/AJPH.2023.307262

ACKNOWLEDGMENTS

I would like to acknowledge and honor my trancestors, both alive and no longer with us on the embodied plane, without whom my existence as a joyful but mad-as-hell transgender person would not be possible. *A luta continua.*

CONFLICTS OF INTEREST

At the time of publication (but not at the time that this opinion piece was solicited), one of the coauthors of the article being reviewed (S. K. Kattari) was a compensated member of B. E. Coston's grant-funded project's community steering committee. To B. E. Coston's knowledge, S. K. Kattari was not aware that this opinion piece was solicited and the two did not speak about it before, during, or after it was written and accepted.

REFERENCES

1. Peitzmeier SM, Malik M, Kattari SK, et al. Intimate partner violence in transgender populations: systematic review and meta-analysis of prevalence and correlates. *Am J Public Health.* 2020;110(9):e1–e14. https://doi.org/10.2105/AJPH.2020.305774
2. Snorton CR. *Black on Both Sides: A Racial History of Trans Identity.* Minneapolis, MN: University of Minnesota Press; 2017.
3. Benjamin H. *The Transsexual Phenomenon.* New York, NY: Julian Press; 1966.
4. Stryker S. Transgender history, homonormativity, and disciplinarity. *Radic Hist Rev.* 2008;2008(100):145–157. https://doi.org/10.1215/01636545-2007-026
5. Beemyn G. A presence in the past: a transgender historiography. *J Womens Hist.* 2013;25(4):113–121. https://doi.org/10.1353/jowh.2013.0062
6. Wilson A. Our coming in stories: Cree identity, body sovereignty and gender self-determination. *Journal of Global Indigeneity.* 2015;1(1):4. https://ro.uow.edu.au/jgi/vol1/iss1/4
7. Alter KJ, Zürn M. Theorising backlash politics: conclusion to a special issue on backlash politics in comparison. *Br J Polit Int Relat.* 2020;22(4):739–752. https://doi.org/10.1177/1369148120947956
8. Bettcher TM. Evil deceivers and make-believers: on transphobic violence and the politics of illusion. *Hypatia.* 2007;22(3):43–65. https://doi.org/10.1111/j.1527-2001.2007.tb01090.x
9. Branigan A, Kirkpatrick N. Anti-trans laws are on the rise. Here's a look at where—and what kind. *Washington Post.* October 14, 2022. Available at: https://www.washingtonpost.com/lifestyle/2022/10/14/anti-trans-bills. Accessed October 20, 2022.
10. American Civil Liberties Union. Legislation affecting LGBTQ rights across the country. Available at: https://www.aclu.org/legislation-affecting-lgbtq-rights-across-country. Accessed October 20, 2022.
11. Human Rights Campaign. Anti-Transgender legislation spreads nationwide, bills targeting transgender children surge. February 19, 2016. Available at: https://assets2.hrc.org/files/assets/resources/HRC-Anti-Trans-Issue-Brief-FINAL-REV2.pdf. Accessed October 20, 2022.
12. National Coalition of Anti-Violence Programs. A crisis of hate: a report on lesbian. gay, bisexual, transgender and queer hate violence homicides in 2017. 2018. Available at: https://antiviolence.wpenginepowered.com/wp-content/uploads/2018/01/a-crisis-of-hate-january-release.pdf. Accessed October 19, 2022.
13. Schmidt S, Mayes BR, Decaille N. Surviving as a Black transgender woman in Baton Rouge. *Washington Post.* June 29, 2021. Available at: https://www.washingtonpost.com/dc-md-va/2021/06/28/transgender-women-homicides-intimate-partner-violence. Accessed October 19, 2022.
14. Raymond JG. Technology on the social and ethical aspects of transsexual surgery. September 16, 2011. Available at: https://www.susans.org/wiki/Technology_on_the_Social_and_Ethical_Aspects_of_Transsexual_Surgery. Accessed October 2, 2022.
15. Malatino H. *Trans Care.* Minneapolis, MN: University of Minnesota Press; 2020.
16. National Sexual Violence Resource Center. Resources and support for transgender survivors. November 21, 2021. Available at: https://www.nsvrc.org/blogs/resources-and-support-transgender-survivors. Accessed October 19, 2022.

Vladeck Redux: Our Endlessly Imperfect American Health Care System

John E. McDonough, DrPH, MPA

ABOUT THE AUTHOR

John E. McDonough is a professor of practice at the Harvard T. H. Chan School of Public Health, Boston, MA.

For years in our modern era, a widely accepted political truism was that no one from either major political party could win the White House without first winning the New Hampshire presidential primary. When Bill Clinton won the White House in 1992 after losing the Granite State primary, the truism was modified to apply only to *Republican* candidates. After George W. Bush did the same in 2000, well, never mind. "It's tough to make predictions, especially about the future," noted Yogi Berra.[1]

Writing this commentary on a 20-year-old article is a guilty pleasure. The pleasure comes from revisiting the ideas of Bruce Vladeck, a health policy legend who ran the US Health Care Financing Administration under President Bill Clinton. He is an indefatigable advocate for disadvantaged groups and for the US health care safety net. His policy writing is always illuminating and indispensable, including for this commentary. The guilty part is identifying mistaken predictions via the sweet, powerful elixir of hindsight. It's just too easy.

Vladeck's 2003 *AJPH* article, "Universal Health Insurance in the United States: Reflections on the Past, the Present, and the Future," offers historical-cultural and structural-political explanations for the United States' lack of universal health insurance.[2] Written in a period of Republican "trifecta" control of the White House, Senate, and House of Representatives, the only viable national health policy aspiration at that time was adding outpatient prescription drug coverage to Medicare, which happened that December in the form of Part D.

At that time, many health policymakers and advocates were still licking their wounds from the 1993–1994 Clinton health reform catastrophe and the 1997 Balanced Budget Act, which had been financed largely by cuts to Medicare. No leading indicator of the future Affordable Care Act, signed in 2010, was visible on the nation's political radar screen. Buying outpatient drugs for Medicare enrollees had been an explicit campaign promise from both 2000 presidential candidates, George W. Bush and Al Gore. Expanding insurance coverage for about 40 million uninsured Americans—universally or incrementally—did not seem to matter as much then.

Many of Vladeck's historical-cultural explanations for the laggard status of US health insurance coverage are spot-on relevant today. These include many Americans' long-standing antipathy toward government, well baked into our political culture. The lack of working-class solidarity, the absence of a national labor party, plus deep and persistent racial divides, all have blocked social progress, he aptly observed. Reinforcing these trends in current time, US union membership continues its decades-long decline, from 20.1% in 1983 to 12.9% in 2003, and to 10.1% in 2022.[3]

Likewise, Vladeck's political-structural explanations remain persuasive. Our enduring Madisonian republic purposefully inhibits "small-d" democratic advances through the division of powers among three federal branches of government and between the two houses of Congress. Achieving substantial social and economic advances is more feasible in parliamentary systems where legislative and executive powers are joined.

As a result, our dispersed public powers and authorities have always been unequal, still true today, although less explicitly than when political power was monopolized well into the 19th century by property-owning White men. The 2011 Occupy Wall Street movement, Thomas Piketty's ground-breaking 2014 book on historic and contemporary income and wealth inequality, and the 2020 Minneapolis, Minnesota murder of George Floyd are three thunderous reminders of how much has not changed and needs action.[4]

Vladeck wrote seven years before the US Supreme Court's 2010 *Citizens United* ruling, which unleashed torrents of unlimited spending on political campaigns by corporations and the wealthy. Even in 2003, he observed how "the power of money becomes

AJPH May 2023, Vol 113, No. 5

even greater . . . political contributions can often be evaluated in terms of simple return on investment. Groups with significant economic resources have long been opposed to universal health insurance."[2(p17)] He—and we—had no idea how much worse campaign finance would become by 2023.

Understandably, not all Vladeck's conclusions hold today—and those also are worth consideration. Vladeck wrote in a period of outspoken despair at endlessly poor prospects for meaningful insurance coverage advances. Yet just seven years later, a Democratic trifecta under President Barack Obama enjoyed a 60-vote filibuster-proof Senate majority for just seven magic months (July 2009 to January 2010) and used that to achieve major expansion and reform via the Affordable Care Act (ACA). Democrats accomplished this with zero Republican support and thus without policy concessions that would have watered down the ACA beyond recognition. Vladeck did not see this coming, and no one else did either.

Context matters in ways not so obvious in 2003. Vladeck wrote in the middle of the nation's 40-year embrace of neoliberal and free-market fundamentalist ideas then holding a tight grip on our body politic. The startling 2008 economic collapse shook Americans' consciousness and delivered control of the White House and Congressional majorities barely sufficient to pass the ACA. Unlike Medicare and Medicaid, created in 1965 by President Lyndon Johnson during the New Deal era, the ACA needed to conform to neoliberal notions that private health insurance was superior to the public brand. Even creating a smallish "public option" in ACA insurance marketplaces was a political bridge too far.

Although neither the 2008–2010 financial collapse nor the ongoing COVID-19 pandemic fomented a full counterrevolution, the ground is shifting today. As Michael Tomasky documents in his 2022 book, *The Middle Out*, widespread public acceptance of tax cuts for the wealthy and deregulation have both lost steam.[5(p13)] Today, a new generation of progressive ideas on government and social policy have taken hold within the Biden Administration, among Congressional Democrats and some Republicans, and in American opinion. Team Biden, especially those in the Federal Trade Commission and the Justice Department, have reenergized aggressive antitrust and antimonopoly enforcement, mostly dormant since the 1970s. Negotiating Medicare drug pricing, 19 years after Part D's creation, is now law and in implementation. Increasing taxes on corporations and the wealthy as well as reversing deregulation are no longer anathema. Times change, and the desultory realities of an earlier era no longer carry the same weight.

Another example worth mulling is Vladeck's assertion that "as a practical matter, you can reform the health care delivery system or you can reform health insurance, but you can't do both at the same time."[2] The ACA became law with provisions to expand and reform health insurance and to reorient the medical care delivery system through a value-based care policy agenda. The latter includes creation of vertically integrated "accountable care organizations," experiments with bundled payment, electronic health records, and much more.

In 2023, those coverage expansions now stand as strong successes, bringing the national uninsured rate down to 8% in 2021, the lowest rate since the United States started counting in the 1960s.[6] Meanwhile, the value-based agenda moves forward, although failing to show meaningful quality improvements in the face of continuing cost increases. Ten years ago, smart money bet on the reverse outcomes—success for value-based care and failure for coverage. Either way, the ACA has demonstrated that walking and chewing gum at the same time can happen.

I end where Vladeck began, with his note that South Africa in 2003 publicly committed to achieving universal health insurance and thus would soon part company with the United States as one of the two industrialized nations without universal coverage. Twenty years on, South Africa has made zero progress toward universal or even greatly expanded coverage. Although the United States has not achieved universal coverage, it has delivered meaningful reform and progress. With the passage of the 2021 American Rescue Plan Act and the 2022 Inflation Reduction Act, that substantial and real progress continues.

Although major challenges persist ahead, including the explosion in medical debt, the increasing and dangerous financialization and corporatization of American medicine, as well as gaping and enduring racial, ethnic, and other health inequities, the commitment and drive of Americans to system reform remains unshakable. AJPH

CORRESPONDENCE

Correspondence should be sent to John E. McDonough, Department of Health Policy & Management, Harvard T.H. Chan School of Public Health, 677 Huntington Ave, Boston, MA 02115 (e-mail: jmcdonough@hsph.harvard.edu). Reprints can be ordered at http://www.ajph.org by clicking the "Reprints" link.

PUBLICATION INFORMATION

Full Citation: McDonough JE. Vladeck redux: our endlessly imperfect American health care system. *Am J Public Health*. 2023;113(5):477–479.

Acceptance Date: February 16, 2023.

DOI: https://doi.org/10.2105/AJPH.2023.307265

CONFLICTS OF INTEREST

The author has no conflicts of interest to disclose.

REFERENCES

1. Liberman M. Linguistic humor, Yogi Berra, sayings and ripostes. Available at: https://www.ling.upenn.edu/~beatrice/humor/yogi-berra.html. Accessed March 4, 2023.
2. Vladeck B. Universal health insurance in the United States: reflections on the past, the present, and the future. *Am J Public Health*. 2003;93(1):16–19. https://doi.org/10.2105/AJPH.93.1.16
3. Bureau of Labor Statistics. Union members—2022. January 19, 2023. Available at: https://www.bls.gov/news.release/pdf/union2.pdf. Accessed March 4, 2023.
4. Piketty T. *Capital in the 21st Century*. Cambridge, MA: Harvard University Press; 2013. https://doi.org/10.4159/9780674369542
5. Tomasky M. *The Middle Out: The Rise of Progressive Economics and a Return to Shared Prosperity*. New York, NY: Doubleday; 2022.
6. Lee A, Ruhter J, Peters C, De Lew N, Sommers BD. National uninsured rate reaches all-time low in early 2022. Office of the Assistant Secretary for Planning and Evaluation, US Dept of Health and Human Services. August 2, 2022. Available at: https://aspe.hhs.gov/reports/2022-uninsurance-at-all-time-low. Accessed March 4, 2023.

Public Health Practice and Health Equity for Vulnerable Workers: A Public Health of Consequence, May 2023

Farzana Kapadia, PhD, MPH

ABOUT THE AUTHOR

Farzana Kapadia is the deputy editor of AJPH *and professor of epidemiology at the School of Global Public Health, New York University, New York, NY.*

See also Porter et al., p. 500.

AJPH May 2023, Vol 113, No. 5

Structured vulnerabilities that threaten the health of meat- and poultry-packing workers are driven by a complex and complicated host of economic, occupational, social, and health care access–related factors. Recognition of these complexities is a first step. More challenging, yet critical to sustaining a commitment to social justice for these frontline workers, are public health practice initiatives rooted in health equity that work toward eliminating health disparities.

In this issue of *AJPH*, Porter et al. (p. 500) describe implementation of a public health practice initiative aimed at reducing COVID-19 vaccine hesitancy and increasing vaccine uptake among poultry industry workers. This editorial seeks to contextualize this initiative as one investment in a larger constellation of investments that are needed to provide resources and services equally to all members of our society.

STRUCTURED VULNERABILITIES AND ESSENTIAL WORKERS

Employees of the meat- and poultry-packing industry are overwhelmingly racialized workers, immigrants, or refugees and more likely to be living in poverty. According to analyses by the Economic Policy Institute, which used 2014–2018 American Community Survey data, animal slaughtering and processing workers were more likely to identify as Black (21.9%), Latinx (34.9%), or Asian (6.8%); to be foreign-born (37.5%); and to live below the poverty line (8.8%) compared with all US workers. By industry, women were more likely to be employed by poultry processing (40.1%) than meatpacking (32.2%) companies (https://bit.ly/3lx3mqC). And largely resulting from historically stronger union activity among meatpacking workers in urban areas, the proportion of poultry-processing workers living below the poverty line is double that among meatpacking workers (11.4% vs 5.6%).

These intersections of race and ethnicity, immigration and citizenship status, low socioeconomic status, and unfair labor policies and practices has had profound implications for the health status of poultry- and meatpacking industry employees. Even before the COVID-19 pandemic, the meat- and poultry-packing industry was one of the most hazardous industries to be employed in in the United States, and a recent report from the National Employment Law Project showed that reports of severe injury were highest among poultry-processing workers (https://bit.ly/3xsd5bH). On top of these preexisting dangerous conditions, the health and safety of meatpacking and poultry-processing employees and their families were further jeopardized when federal mandates during the COVID-19 pandemic were issued rendering these employees as essential workers.

Efforts to protect meat and poultry industry workers during the early stages of the pandemic were, at best, inconsistently applied as protective measures were deemed guidance rather than mandatory requirements. Forced to work under already dangerous conditions, workers continued in unsafe and unsanitary conditions without necessary personal protective equipment, ability to physically or socially distance, or granted paid time off for sick leave. According to data collected by the Food and Environment Reporting Network, between March 1, 2020, and September 2, 2021, 1466 meatpacking and food-processing plants reported confirmed COVID-19 cases where more than 90 000 workers had tested positive for COVID-19 and 466 workers died (https://bit.ly/3lLSJr0). These numbers are still considered underestimates as COVID-19 cases may have been missed or untested, especially among undocumented workers who are less likely to seek testing and care for fear of deportation.

COVID-19 VACCINE EQUITY FOR ESSENTIAL WORKERS

According to the US Bureau of Labor Statistics, Arkansas ranks just below Georgia with the second-highest number of workers employed in the poultry-processing industry. Recognizing that targeting COVID-19 vaccination efforts to an already vulnerable population that comprises a substantial portion of the population can reduce COVID-19 cases at the community level as well, the Arkansas Department of Health launched the Joining Forces for Better Health initiative. The initiative included vaccine education videos in Spanish and Marshallese and vaccination programs implemented in collaboration with poultry- and meat-packing companies in the state. Powers et al. provide evidence that this effort, specifically designed to increase accessibility to COVID-19 vaccines at worksites for employees as well as their family members, allowed for vaccines to be delivered in these settings.

EQUITY IN PUBLIC HEALTH PRACTICE

Echoing previous work,[1] these findings support the need for greater and continued investment in vaccination and primary care programs that work with community members to provide culturally relevant and linguistically appropriate information as an equity approach for workers engaged in high-risk environments and occupations, particularly those in rural settings. However, on their own, these programs are insufficient to reduce disease risk and improve population health outcomes.

First, recognizing that workers in these industries are impacted by multiple unjust labor practices including job insecurity, inadequate health insurance, low wages, and lack of paid sick-leave calls for prioritizing fair and equitable employment practices for these frontline workers. Second, regulations that improve workplace safety standards and provide durable and high-quality protective equipment to all workers will certainly enhance worker safety.[2,3] Third, given that undocumented immigrants constitute a large proportion of frontline workers in the meatpacking and poultry-processing industries, states and counties with large proportions of undocumented immigrants must enhance policies and practices that protect as well as support this marginalized group.[4,5] Finally, multisector approaches to improving the social conditions of workers by providing access to affordable and safe housing to living in substandard and crowded housing conditions, having limited transportation options, and experiences of discrimination and stigma because of race, ethnicity, immigration status, and gender shape population health outcomes. Working across sectors and providing a comprehensive, societal approach will surely yield greater population health impacts. AJPH

CORRESPONDENCE

Correspondence should be sent to Farzana Kapadia, PhD, MPH, New York University, School of Global Public Health, 708 Broadway, Room 729, New York, NY 10003 (e-mail: farzana.kapadia@nyu.edu). Reprints can be ordered at https://ajph.org by clicking the "Reprints" link.

PUBLICATION INFORMATION

Full Citation: Kapadia F. Public health practice and health equity for vulnerable workers: a public health of consequence, May 2023. *Am J Public Health*. 2023;113(5):480–481.

Acceptance Date: February 18, 2023.

DOI: https://doi.org/10.2105/AJPH.2023.307268

CONFLICTS OF INTEREST

The author has no conflicts of interest to disclose.

REFERENCES

1. Casey MM, Blewett LA, Call KT. Providing health care to Latino immigrants: community-based efforts in the rural Midwest. *Am J Public Health*. 2004;94(10):1709–1711. https://doi.org/10.2105/AJPH.94.10.1709
2. Seminario MM. The Occupational Safety and Health Act at 50—a labor perspective. *Am J Public Health*. 2020;110(5):642–643. https://doi.org/10.2105/AJPH.2019.305541
3. Azaroff LS, Levenstein C, Wegman DH. Occupational injury and illness surveillance: conceptual filters explain underreporting. *Am J Public Health*. 2002;92(9):1421–1429. https://doi.org/10.2105/AJPH.92.9.1421
4. DeGarmo E, Rosen J, Rutkow L. Use of law by US states during the COVID-19 pandemic with respect to people who were undocumented. *Am J Public Health*. 2022;112(12):1757–1764. https://doi.org/10.2105/AJPH.2022.307090
5. Bustamante AV, Nwadiuko J, Ortega AN. State-level legislation during the COVID-19 pandemic to offset the exclusion of undocumented immigrants from federal relief efforts. *Am J Public Health*. 2022;112(12):1729–1731. https://doi.org/10.2105/AJPH.2022.307130

Medicaid Expansion: The Unfinished Promise of the Affordable Care Act

Sanjay Kishore, MD, Micah Johnson, MD, and Sara Rosenbaum, JD

ABOUT THE AUTHORS

Sanjay Kishore is a physician at the Equal Justice Initiative and assistant professor at the University of Alabama at Birmingham (Montgomery Campus). Micah Johnson is a resident physician at Brigham and Women's Hospital, Boston, MA. Sara Rosenbaum is a professor of health policy and law at George Washington University, Washington, DC.

AJPH May 2023, Vol 113, No. 5

More than a decade after the Affordable Care Act (ACA) was signed into law, its core promise—guaranteeing health coverage for the poorest Americans in all states—remains to be realized.

MEDICAID EXPANSION LANDSCAPE

The ACA intended to expand Medicaid to the lowest-income individuals across the country, but in 2012 the Supreme Court ruled mandatory expansion unconstitutional and instead left the decision to each individual state. This was a straightforward choice for most states. Medicaid expansion improves access to care, offers financial security for families, and reduces mortality for some conditions.[1] It also draws billions of dollars in revenue to states because the federal government subsidizes 90% of the cost of expansion.

However, as of winter 2023, 11 states continue to refuse Medicaid expansion. In many of these states, traditional Medicaid eligibility standards are extremely restrictive. In Alabama, for instance, parents can only qualify for Medicaid if household incomes are less than 18% of the federal poverty level (less than $4145 annually for a family of three). In 10 states that have refused expansion, working-age adults who are not parents of minor children, not pregnant, and not living with a major disability are locked out of the program completely.

More than 2 million Americans currently live in this "coverage gap": too poor to qualify for subsidized private health insurance but not poor enough to qualify for Medicaid. Because nonexpansion states are disproportionately located in the South, the burden of this decision falls most heavily on people of color; nearly 60% of those in the coverage gap identify as Black or Latino.[2]

The federal government has tried incremental interventions. The American Rescue Plan increased the ACA's already-generous financial incentives to support state expansion, but this further sweetener produced no result. While the House of Representatives passed Build Back Better legislation that extended the private health insurance subsidy system to all people in the coverage gap, this was ultimately scrapped from the Inflation Reduction Act over concerns of cost and rewarding states who chose not to expand Medicaid.

STATUS OF STATE ACTION

Without a federal remedy, what are the prospects for state action? Broadly, change could come either from state governments or ballot referendums. Among state governments, there appears to be legislative momentum in North Carolina.

The two chambers of the North Carolina legislature each passed separate Medicaid expansion bills before adjourning for the summer. A barrier to reconciliation of these bills has been the support of state hospitals; some lawmakers had been calling for reform to the certificate of need policies, which determine which medical services can be offered at certain facilities. Hospitals have been opposed to reforms that might increase competition and decrease revenue, but recently have agreed to these reforms and to help subsidize the state expenses associated with Medicaid expansion. It appears a compromise bill is in sight, a surprising reversal for the Republican-controlled branch where leaders had adamantly opposed expansion, seemingly spurred by the stimulus of federal funds.

In Georgia, Medicaid expansion was a key topic in the gubernatorial race, with Democratic candidate Stacey Abrams arguing that recent hospital closures are attributable to the failure of incumbent Republican Governor Brian Kemp to expand Medicaid, but legislative action is not clear.

The addition of work requirements is a complicating factor. North Carolina's legislation initially but no longer included a compulsory work rule to be eligible for Medicaid; the Centers for Medicare and Medicaid Services (CMS) withdrew previously granted waivers to states like South Carolina and Georgia that allowed work requirements within Medicaid.

This action signals that CMS is not willing to allow states to tether Medicaid expansion to a harmful policy, as demonstrated by a landmark study that showed that work requirements in Arkansas's Medicaid program were associated with losses in health coverage without any significant gains in employment, mostly because of confusion about reporting requirements.[3] The prospects for significant legislative progress on Medicaid expansion among holdout states may be dependent on the federal government's tolerance of work requirements.

The majority of states that have adopted Medicaid expansion after 2019 have done so by ballot referendums; these include Idaho, Maine, Missouri, Nebraska, and Oklahoma. Many of these ballot measures include explicit language prohibiting the addition of other restrictions on eligibility (such as work requirements). South Dakota most recently approved a constitutional amendment guaranteeing Medicaid expansion via ballot referendum in November 2022.[4]

However, among the remaining holdout states, only Florida and Wyoming have broad policies that allow voter referendums. The status of initiatives in these states is unclear; in Florida, an effort to put Medicaid expansion on the ballot was held back by its organizing committee in 2020 after the state legislature raised the number of signatures needed for review. Organizers in Mississippi did successfully petition for a Medicaid expansion ballot initiative that was approved by the Secretary of State in 2021; however, the state Supreme Court later ruled that the state's ballot process was unworkable and inoperative, thereby halting the effort. Alabama, Georgia, Kansas, Tennessee, Texas, and Wisconsin lack a voter-driven ballot initiative process.[5]

The Affordable Care Act was designed to expand access to care to the poorest Americans. However, 12 years later, the refusal to expand Medicaid remains the most potent symbol of political resistance to government's role in health policy and the effort to promote health equity. While there is some momentum around expansion within state governments, this seems to be tied to eligibility restrictions that will compromise access to care. At the same time, many holdout states lack a mechanism for voter-driven referendums to guarantee expansion without these burdens. While there are important opportunities to make progress at the state level, it is likely that congressional action will be necessary to secure universal health coverage for the poorest Americans. AJPH

CORRESPONDENCE

Correspondence should be sent to Sanjay Kishore, MD, 3202 Montezuma Rd, Montgomery, AL 36104 (e-mail: sanjaykishore31@gmail.com). Reprints can be ordered at https://ajph.org by clicking the "Reprints" link.

PUBLICATION INFORMATION

Full Citation: Kishore S, Johnson M, Rosenbaum S. Medicaid expansion: the unfinished promise of the Affordable Care Act. *Am J Public Health.* 2023; 113(5):482–483.

Acceptance Date: February 4, 2023.

DOI: https://doi.org/10.2105/AJPH.2023.307258

CONTRIBUTORS

All authors contributed to the drafting of this editorial.

CONFLICTS OF INTEREST

The authors have no conflicts of interest to disclose.

REFERENCES

1. Lam MB, Phelan J, Orav EJ. Medicaid expansion and mortality among patients with breast, lung, and colorectal cancer. *JAMA Netw Open.* 2020;3(11):e2024366. https://doi.org/10.1001/jamanetworkopen.2020.24366
2. Lukens G, Sharer B. Closing Medicaid coverage gap would help diverse group and narrow racial disparities. Center on Budget and Policy Priorities. Available at: https://www.cbpp.org/research/health/closing-medicaid-coverage-gap-would-help-diverse-group-and-narrow-racial. Accessed August 8, 2022.
3. Sommers BD, Goldman AL, Blendon RJ, Orav EJ, Epstein AM. Medicaid work requirements—results from the first year in Arkansas. *N Engl J Med.* 2019; 381(11):1073–1082. https://doi.org/10.1056/NEJMsr1901772
4. Kaiser Family Foundation. Status of state Medicaid expansion decisions: interactive map. July 21, 2022. Available at: https://www.kff.org/medicaid/issue-brief/status-of-state-medicaid-expansion-decisions-interactive-map. Accessed August 8, 2022.
5. Brantley E, Rosenbaum S. Ballot initiatives have brought Medicaid eligibility to many but cannot solve the coverage gap. *Health Affairs Forefront.* June 23, 2021. Available at: https://www.healthaffairs.org/do/10.1377/forefront.20210617.992286/full. Accessed August 8, 2022.

Government Investment in the Marijuana Industry's Commercial Interests Harms Vulnerable Groups

Linda Richter, PhD, Robyn Oster, BA, and Lindsey Vuolo, JD, MPH

ABOUT THE AUTHORS

All authors are with the Partnership to End Addiction, New York, NY.

AJPH May 2023, Vol 113, No. 5

In designing drug reform laws, we must ensure that efforts to help communities adversely affected by criminalization do not inadvertently inflict further harm on vulnerable populations, including youths and communities of color. Drug reform certainly presents a crucial opportunity to end the disproportionate damage that the War on Drugs inflicted on people of color and economically disadvantaged communities (e.g., higher arrest and incarceration rates; barriers to employment, housing, education, and public benefits; punitive child welfare system involvement).[1] However, we have repeatedly seen how industries selling addictive substances that are legal for adult use (e.g., alcohol, cigarettes, vaping products) target both youths and disadvantaged communities through their product design, marketing, and locations of sale, largely ignoring the outsized negative health and social costs of commercialized addictive substances to these groups.[2,3]

A recent study found that the largest marijuana companies engage in "corporate social responsibility" activities that mimic those the tobacco industry uses to influence politics and regulation, encourage increased consumption, and target marginalized communities.[4] The companies claim that their activities will mitigate the harms of prohibition and promote diversity. The study also reports that marijuana companies assist social equity license applicants in exchange for control of their proposed businesses. These companies are using strategies much like those tobacco companies have used for decades to normalize the use of the substance, recruit new and loyal customers, encourage consumption, expand markets, and deter regulation. Although their stated purpose might appear beneficial, the consequences of their involvement can disproportionately harm the communities they claim to be helping.

The United States is at risk for repeating past mistakes by allowing the marijuana industry, which now includes many of the same players as the alcohol and tobacco industries, to target youths, low-income groups, and communities of color, this time under the guise of social and economic justice.[4,5] Contributing to this phenomenon, several well-intentioned government laws and proposals are creating initiatives and committing resources that support the industry's financial interests, potentially to the detriment of the groups they are purporting to serve.

For example, New York State recently announced $5 million for its public community colleges to support courses and credentialing programs aimed at promoting employment in the emerging cannabis industry.[6] Illinois similarly created its Community College Cannabis Vocational Pilot Program.[7] Although an increasing number of private and public colleges and universities now offer cannabis training programs (focusing on agriculture and horticulture, cannabis-based medicine, and the business of cannabis), these appear to be the first instances of states directly authorizing, funding, and promoting such programs and doing so in schools that primarily serve socioeconomically disadvantaged communities.

RISKS TO YOUTHS

Marijuana legalization, which in the United States invariably takes the form of commercialization, normalizes use among youths, reduces perceptions of harm, and is associated with higher rates of use,[8] especially among young adults for whom rates just reached historic highs.[9] Contrary to the common belief that marijuana's adverse effects primarily pertain to adolescents, research shows significant risks to young people well into early adulthood.[10] Most college students are younger than 21 years, the legal age to purchase marijuana in every state that has legalized adult use of the drug. State-funded school programs encouraging employment in the industry can further normalize use and sale in a population highly vulnerable to its harms. Underage youths who work in the industry also have increased exposure and access to the drug, increasing their risk of frequent use and adverse consequences.[5]

RISKS TO DISADVANTAGED COMMUNITIES

The tobacco and alcohol industries have consistently concentrated their retail outlets in low-income communities and communities of color,[3] much to the detriment of those who live in those areas. Marijuana retail has similarly been concentrated in neighborhoods with lower incomes and higher proportions of racial/ethnic minority populations.[11] Further incentivizing cannabis business development in these communities threatens to target neighborhoods in which the retail and advertising presence of commercialized addictive substances already far exceeds that of less disadvantaged communities.[3]

Federal and state attempts to build employment opportunities for those from historically underserved communities, although laudable, run counter to efforts to address substance use and addiction among at-risk populations. The federal Cannabis Administration and Opportunity Act proposed in 2022 to decriminalize, regulate, and tax marijuana at the federal level, includes provisions that would provide funding to implement cannabis licensing programs that minimize barriers for individuals disproportionately and adversely affected by criminalization, as well as loans and technical assistance to small businesses owned and controlled by socially and economically disadvantaged individuals. Although the bill did not advance in Congress, many states have included similar provisions in their legalization laws. Illinois's community college program, for example, specifically prioritizes schools with student populations that are more than 50% low income.[7]

We have already seen how many well-intentioned social equity programs implemented by states as they legalize marijuana have failed to meet their potential,[12] suggesting that alternative tactics that go beyond promoting involvement in the cannabis industry to redress historical inequities are needed.

Encouraging disadvantaged populations most harmed by inequitable drug laws to engage with an industry promoting a commercialized addictive product through training programs for public college students may run counter to the goals of achieving racial and economic justice.

RECOMMENDATIONS TO MINIMIZE HARM

To help communities that the criminalization of marijuana possession and use has undeniably targeted and harmed, government resources should be allocated to services that mitigate the consequences of those injustices (e.g., through expungement, reentry services, legal aid, job training, small business grants) rather than to assisting a profit-driven industry to sell its product to those same communities.

It is difficult to determine the nature and quality of the courses and programs springing up at hundreds of US colleges across states with different marijuana laws. Given the unique harm that marijuana poses to youths and the general lack of awareness of these adverse effects, states that do authorize and fund college training programs for the cannabis industry should at a minimum ensure key safeguards, including requiring (1) that students be 21 years or older to participate, (2) a course in the curriculum that educates students about the adverse effects of marijuana, (3) input from substance use experts to ensure that the curriculum includes information on protecting underage youths and disadvantaged communities from unscrupulous sales and marketing strategies, and (4) equal or greater funding for marijuana use prevention and mitigation efforts.

We know from experience with the tobacco and alcohol industries that when they are involved in school-based programs, those programs frequently do more to normalize and promote substance use than to protect students from those substances. Those industries' lobbying efforts and purported attempts to benefit society have been proven to contradict their stated goals, instead serving to boost their profits, not public health. With these same industries increasingly involved in marijuana commercialization, protecting public health should be government's main focus.

One stated goal of the Cannabis Administration and Opportunity Act is to regulate marijuana with a framework similar to that for alcohol and tobacco. Governments have never explicitly promoted alcohol and tobacco businesses, nor should it encourage marijuana commerce through college training programs. The decriminalization of marijuana use and possession is critical and must be accompanied by smart policies to remedy past and ongoing inequities. Governments should fund services and programs to promote employment and redress these injustices without promoting the industry that is commercializing an addictive substance, inevitably to the harm of youths and disadvantaged communities. AJPH

CORRESPONDENCE

Correspondence should be sent to Linda Richter, Partnership to End Addiction, 711 Third Ave, 5th Floor, Suite 500, New York, NY 10017 (e-mail: lrichter@toendaddiction.org). Reprints can be ordered at http://www.ajph.org by clicking the "Reprints" link.

PUBLICATION INFORMATION

Full Citation: Richter L, Oster R, Vuolo L. Government investment in the marijuana industry's commercial interests harms vulnerable groups. *Am J Public Health*. 2023;113(5):484–486.

Acceptance Date: February 4, 2023.

DOI: https://doi.org/10.2105/AJPH.2023.307257

CONTRIBUTORS

All authors contributed to conceptualizing, drafting, and revising this editorial and approved the final version.

CONFLICTS OF INTEREST

The authors have no potential or actual conflicts of interest to disclose.

REFERENCES

1. Cohen A, Vakharia SP, Netherland J, Frederique K. How the war on drugs impacts social determinants of health beyond the criminal legal system. *Ann Med*. 2022;54(1):2024–2038. https://doi.org/10.1080/07853890.2022.2100926
2. Kirchner TR, Villanti AC, Cantrell J, et al. Tobacco retail outlet advertising practices and proximity to schools, parks and public housing affect Synar underage sales violations in Washington, DC. *Tob Control*. 2015;24(suppl 1):e52–e58. https://doi.org/10.1136/tobaccocontrol-2013-051239
3. Wheeler DC, Boyle J, Barsell DJ, et al. Associations of alcohol and tobacco retail outlet rates with neighborhood disadvantage. *Int J Environ Res Public Health*. 2022;19(3):1134. https://doi.org/10.3390/ijerph19031134
4. Wakefield T, Glantz SA, Apollonio DE. Content analysis of the corporate social responsibility practices of 9 major cannabis companies in Canada and the US. *JAMA Netw Open*. 2022;5(8):e2228088. https://doi.org/10.1001/jamanetworkopen.2022.28088
5. Sabet K. Smokescreen: what the marijuana industry doesn't want you to know. *Mo Med*. 2021;118(5):411–415. https://www.ncbi.nlm.nih.gov/pmc/articles/PMC8504499/#_ffn_sectitle
6. Governor of New York. Governor Hochul announces $5 million in funding to support the launch of new and existing cannabis accreditation programs. July 18, 2022. Available at: https://www.governor.ny.gov/news/governor-hochul-announces-5-million-funding-support-launch-new-and-existing-cannabis. Accessed November 17, 2022.
7. Cannabis Regulation and Tax Act. 410 Ill. Comp. Stat. 705/(2019).
8. Committee on Substance Abuse, Committee on Adolescence. The impact of marijuana policies on youth: clinical, research, and legal update. *Pediatrics*. 2015;135(3):584–587. https://doi.org/10.1542/peds.2014-4146.
9. University of Michigan. Marijuana, hallucinogen use at all-time high among young adults. Michigan News. August 22, 2022. Available at: https://news.umich.edu/marijuana-hallucinogen-use-at-all-time-high-among-young-adults. Accessed November 17, 2022.
10. Richter L. The prevention of nonmedical marijuana use must extend past adolescence. *J Adolesc Health*. 2022;71(1):6–7. https://doi.org/10.1016/j.jadohealth.2022.04.002
11. Shi Y, Meseck K, Jankowska MM. Availability of medical and recreational marijuana stores and neighborhood characteristics in Colorado. *J Addict*. 2016;2016:7193740. https://doi.org/10.1155/2016/7193740
12. Gerber M. California promised "social equity" after pot legalization. Those hit hardest feel betrayed. *Los Angeles Times*. January 27, 2022. Available at: https://www.latimes.com/california/story/2022-01-27/california-pot-industry-social-equity-broken-promises. Accessed November 17, 2022.

Cannabis Equity Initiatives: Progress, Problems, and Potentials

Y. Tony Yang, ScD, LLM, MPH, Carla J. Berg, PhD, MBA, and Scott Burris, JD

ABOUT THE AUTHORS

Y. Tony Yang is with School of Nursing, Milken Institute School of Public Health, GW Cancer Center, the George Washington University, Washington, DC. Carla J. Berg is with Milken Institute School of Public Health, GW Cancer Center, the George Washington University. Scott Burris is with the Center for Public Health Law Research at the Beasley School of Law, Temple University, Philadelphia, PA.

As of November 9, 2022, 37 states and the District of Columbia have authorized medical cannabis, 21 of which also authorized recreational cannabis.[1] The ongoing dismantling of cannabis "prohibition" follows public opinion expressed in polls and ballot initiatives.[2] While it also reflects the failure of criminalization as a mechanism to regulate cannabis, experience with alcohol and tobacco shows that public health law can and should play a powerful role in minimizing harms to health and civility.[3]

Of all the regulatory challenges posed by a burgeoning industry, none has greater moral weight than addressing racial inequities caused by cannabis regulation. Prohibition of cannabis had more roots in racism than epidemiology.[4] Despite roughly equal usage rates, Blacks are 3.73 times more likely than Whites to be arrested for cannabis possession, suffering both the individual and community harms of criminal justice involvement.[5] Even today, as the cannabis industry transitions from criminal enterprise to legal business, inequities persist with more than 80% of cannabis business owners being White.[6] Society has an opportunity now to ensure that a fair proportion of the benefits of the new industry accrue to individuals and communities harmed by prohibition. Recent legalization efforts try to address these disparities through social and economic equity requirements; however, clear and reproducible efficacy remains to be seen. This commentary discusses three major governmental approaches to accomplish this, along with their problems and potentials.

EXPUNGEMENT OF PAST CONVICTIONS

A drug-related criminal record carries life-long consequences, affecting the convicted person's employment opportunities, eligibility for loans, rental options, and child custody, for example. Most states prohibit people with prior drug felonies from becoming cannabis business owners or serving in other leadership roles, blocking their entry into the industry.

In October 2022, President Biden issued a blanket pardon of federal convictions for simple cannabis possession.[7] Twenty-one states have enacted legislation explicitly permitting or facilitating the process of having select cannabis convictions expunged, vacated, or otherwise sealed from public view.[8] While some states (e.g., Illinois, Vermont, New York) have local jurisdictions automatically perform the review and expungement process, other states require that those with past convictions actively petition their officials for an expungement.[8]

These actions are helpful, but clearing a criminal record for possession of cannabis does not redress missed economic, educational, and social opportunities. It does nothing for people who also have convictions for other minor drug possession felonies or who were also charged as dealers. Yet, the logic of addressing the harms of criminalization and overincarceration—and the practicalities of removing the burdens a record places on socioeconomic reintegration—apply to these convictions as well: a person whose record included convictions for cocaine or illicit opioid possession will still be subject to the same legal disabilities, including a ban from working in the cannabis industry, no matter how long ago or minor their crime was.

In a context of large-scale criminalization of lower-income Black people, removing one conviction will not have a significant population effect. There are at least two ways to better redress the harms of failed drug policies and curtail future harms. The first is to extend pardons and expungement to all crimes of simple possession under controlled substances law and to follow Oregon's lead by eliminating future criminal penalties for simple drug possession.[9] Oregon reclassified personal possession of small amounts of drugs from a Class A misdemeanor to no more than a violation; instead of arrest, possession results in either a $100 fine or a health assessment, including substance use disorder screening.[9]

AJPH May 2023, Vol 113, No. 5

The second is to systematically remove state and federal postconviction socioeconomic limitations and disabilities; this would allow currently law-abiding people with past drug convictions to enter the cannabis business and foster their reintegration into their communities. These remedies provide critical relief by eliminating the stigmatizing record and, as a result, greatly reduce the collateral consequences associated with previous unjust enforcement.

LICENSING AND EMPLOYMENT PREFERENCES

Several cannabis equity programs include a preferential licensure scheme to benefit businesses with owners from marginalized communities negatively impacted by the War on Drugs. Oakland, California, for example, sets aside half of its cannabis business permits for equity applicants who are city residents with an annual income of 80% or less than the city's median and who were either arrested or convicted for cannabis-related crime in the city or lived 10 out of the last 20 years in historically overpoliced areas.[10] The scheme avoids race as a criterion and any mention of a "quota," sidestepping strict limits on affirmative action in racial matters set by the Supreme Court.[11] By contrast, two courts struck down Ohio's 2016 licensing system specifying that 15% of its licenses be granted to racial minorities, stating that it violated the Equal Protection Clause.[12]

States with these programs require (or permit) applicants to include a diversity or social equity plan in their applications. Once they receive these plans, the states add additional application points to an applicant's "score" depending on qualifiers including an applicant's previous cannabis arrests, convictions, or adjudications, as well as their residency; income; racial, cultural, or ethnic background; and if they are female or a veteran. Some states consider additional factors—for instance, whether the majority of employees live in designated disadvantaged areas or the extent of the diverse business owners' ownership and control.

Equity initiatives also address staffing. Oakland, for example, requires that at least half of a dispensary's staff be city residents, half of whom must be from lower-income sections of the city.[10] Advocates argue that residency requirements are necessary to ensure that residents reap the benefits of legalization, but such requirements also face legal challenges. In Detroit, Michigan, a policy allocating 50% of licenses to entrepreneurs who satisfied a residency requirement with social equity components was struck down as a likely violation of the Dormant Commerce Clause, which forbids state laws that interfere with interstate commerce.[13]

Preferential licensing programs have unfortunately not demonstrated significant success. In New York State, half of all cannabis licenses are designated for social equity applicants, but in 2019, only two social equity applicants were approved.[14] In Massachusetts, only 27 out of 122 applicants were given priority by regulators in 2018, and only eight of those received licenses.[15] This is not surprising. By some estimates, starting a cannabis business requires at least \$250 000 in capital for fees, licensure, and other requirements, combined with atypical security and operating costs.[16] Because cannabis remains federally illegal, banks are unable to grant typical business loans to start-ups, and equity entrepreneurs must compete with more established, well-resourced players, potentially increasing predatory business practices.[17] Legal limitations and the momentum of market developments severely restrict the capacity of states and cities to influence the composition of the cannabis ownership class, which is now dominated by White business owners and larger cannabis companies.

TAX REVENUE FOR EQUITY

Some state and local programs require governmental reinvestments of cannabis-related tax revenue into disproportionately impacted communities. This varies significantly by program, but typically includes directed grant programs. For example, in New York State, 40% of cannabis tax revenue funds education, mental health services, substance abuse treatment, and economic development grants.[18] In Portland, Oregon, its 3% cannabis sales tax funds business development and social justice program grants.[18] In California, cannabis tax revenue funds grants to disadvantaged communities, with 50% dedicated to local nonprofits.[18] In Illinois, 25% of cannabis tax revenue must fund grants for violence prevention, reentry, youth development, economic development, or legal aid services.[18]

Taxes can generate significant funding. In California, for example, grants are expected to reach \$50 million in 2023.[19] Moreover, long-term, consistent funding for community programs holds promise for addressing the harms of both drugs and drug prohibition. A hypothetical analysis suggested that earmarking a quarter of cannabis tax revenue could improve structural determinants of mental health among Black and Hispanic communities.[20] In Washington, for example, this would add $117 million a year to the state's mental health budget, increasing it by an estimated 11%.[20] However, grant programs generally have high upkeep costs and are limited in their potential impact on the basis of the performance of individual grantees and duration of funding. In addition, there is always the concern that dedicated funds will replace, rather than supplement, traditional appropriations.

CONCLUSION

Addressing past harms of the War on Drugs relies on serious ongoing efforts, informed by past and current experiences as policies evolve. Currently, state and local cannabis equity legislation lacks substance, in part because of insufficient attention to—and research about—how these policies are implemented and evolving, and their limited impact so far. While clearing criminal records of cannabis possession convictions benefits a few in terms of redressing prohibition's harms, a serious attempt at undoing the harms of prohibition would encompass all low-level drug possession records. Affirmative action in the licensing and operation of cannabis businesses could be a powerful form of redress, but the current Supreme Court majority has signaled opposition to race-conscious policies.[21] Regardless, equity programs do not address the economic challenges to entering the industry. Dedicating cannabis tax revenue to community reinvestment in places historically harmed by prohibition is perhaps the most promising approach, but it depends on enough money being sent to the right recipients for a sufficient number of years. AJPH

CORRESPONDENCE

Correspondence should be sent to Y. Tony Yang, 1919 Pennsylvania Ave NW, Ste 500, Washington, DC 20006 (e-mail: ytyang@gwu.edu). Reprints can be ordered at https://ajph.org by clicking the "Reprints" link.

PUBLICATION INFORMATION

Full Citation: Yang YT, Berg CJ, Burris S. Cannabis equity initiatives: progress, problems, and potentials. *Am J Public Health*. 2023;113(5):487–489.

Acceptance Date: February 8, 2023.

DOI: https://doi.org/10.2105/AJPH.2023.307255

CONTRIBUTORS

Y. T. Yang drafted the article. C. J. Berg and S. Burris revised it critically for important intellectual content.

ACKNOWLEDGMENTS

This article is supported by a grant from the National Institute on Drug Abuse, National Institutes of Health (R01DA054751; MPIs: Berg, Cavazos-Rehg).

CONFLICTS OF INTEREST

The authors have no conflicts of interest.

REFERENCES

1. National Conference of State Legislatures. Cannabis overview. Available at: https://www.ncsl.org/health/state-medical-cannabis-laws. Accessed January 23, 2023.
2. Pew Research Center. Americans overwhelmingly say marijuana should be legal for recreational or medical use. April 16, 2021. Available at: https://www.pewresearch.org/fact-tank/2021/04/16/americans-overwhelmingly-say-marijuana-should-be-legal-for-recreational-or-medical-use. Accessed October 24, 2022.
3. Pacula RL, Kilmer B, Wagenaar AC, Chaloupka FJ, Caulkins JP. Developing public health regulations for marijuana: lessons from alcohol and tobacco. *Am J Public Health*. 2014;104(6):1021–1028. https://doi.org/10.2105/AJPH.2013.301766
4. Solomon R. Racism and its effect on cannabis research. *Cannabis Cannabinoid Res*. 2020;5(1):2–5. https://doi.org/10.1089/can.2019.0063
5. American Civil Liberties Union. A tale of two countries: racially targeted arrests in the era of marijuana reform. 2020. Available at: https://www.aclusd.org/en/marijuana-report. Accessed October 24, 2022.
6. McVey E. Chart: Percentage of cannabis business owners and founders by race. *MJBizDaily*. Available at: https://mjbizdaily.com/chart-19-cannabis-businesses-owned-founded-racial-minorities. Accessed October 24, 2022.
7. The White House. A proclamation on granting pardon for the offense of simple possession of marijuana. October 6, 2022. Available at: https://www.whitehouse.gov/briefing-room/presidential-actions/2022/10/06/granting-pardon-for-the-offense-of-simple-possession-of-marijuana. Accessed October 24, 2022.
8. Collateral Consequences Resource Center. 50-state comparison: marijuana legalization, decriminalization, expungement, and clemency. Available at: https://ccresourcecenter.org/state-restoration-profiles/50-state-comparison-marijuana-legalization-expungement. Accessed October 24, 2022.
9. Oregon State Legislature. Measure 110 (2020). Available at: https://www.oregonlegislature.gov/lpro/Publications/Background-Brief-Measure-110-(2020).pdf. Accessed October 24, 2022.
10. The City of Oakland. Cannabis Equity Program. Available at: https://www.oaklandca.gov/topics/equity-program. Accessed October 24, 2022.
11. *Adarand Constructors Inc v. Peña*, 515 US 200 (1995).
12. *PharmaCann Ohio LLC v. Ohio Department of Commerce* (Ohio Com Pl 2018).
13. *Lowe v. City of Detroit* (ED Mich 2021).
14. New York State, Office of Cannabis Management. What is in the law: social and economic equity. Available at: https://cannabis.ny.gov/system/files/documents/2022/02/cannabis-management-fact-sheet-social-equity_0_0.pdf. Accessed October 24, 2022.
15. Quinton S. Black-owned pot businesses remain rare despite diversity efforts. January 15, 2021. The Pew Charitable Trusts. Available at: https://www.pewtrusts.org/en/research-and-analysis/blogs/stateline/2021/01/15/black-owned-pot-businesses-remain-rare-despite-diversity-efforts. Accessed October 24, 2022.
16. Moore B. How much does it actually cost to open a dispensary? The National Cannabis Industry Association. September 25, 2018. Available at: https://thecannabisindustry.org/member-blog-how-much-does-it-actually-cost-to-open-a-dispensary. Accessed October 24, 2022.
17. Naeem KF. Local cannabis collective recommends changes to Long Beach's failing Cannabis Social Equity Program. *Signal Tribune*. July 26, 2021. Available at: https://sigtrib.com/local-cannabis-collective-recommends-changes-to-long-beachs-failing-cannabis-social-equity-program. Accessed January 23, 2023.
18. The Marijuana Policy Project. Cannabis tax revenue in states that regulate cannabis for adult use. Available at: https://www.mpp.org/issues/legalization/cannabis-tax-revenue-states-regulate-cannabis-adult-use. Accessed October 24, 2022.
19. State of California. California Community Reinvestment Grants Program. Available at: https://business.ca.gov/california-community-reinvestment-grants-program. Accessed October 24, 2022.
20. Purtle J, Brinson K, Stadnick NA. Earmarking excise taxes on recreational cannabis for investments in mental health: an underused financing strategy. *JAMA Health Forum*. 2022;3(4):e220292. https://doi.org/10.1001/jamahealthforum.2022.0292
21. The Supreme Court of the United States. *Students For Fair Admissions Inc v. President and Fellows of Harvard College*. October 31, 2022. Available at: https://www.supremecourt.gov/oral_arguments/argument_transcripts/2022/20-1199_6537.pdf. Accessed January 23, 2023.

Returns to Homelessness: Key Considerations for Using This Metric to Improve System Performance

Jack Tsai, PhD, MSCP, and Thomas Byrne, PhD

ABOUT THE AUTHORS

Both authors are with the US Department of Veterans Affairs National Center on Homelessness Among Veterans, Washington, DC. Jack Tsai is also with the School of Public Health, University of Texas Health Science Center at Houston. Tom Byrne is also with the School of Social Work, Boston University, Boston, MA.

AJPH May 2023, Vol 113, No. 5

In many health care and social service fields, considerable attention is paid to primary prevention (i.e., preventing a condition before it occurs) and secondary prevention (i.e., identifying and treating a condition as soon as possible after it occurs). However, tertiary prevention—defined as managing a condition after it has occurred or preventing recurrence—is a crucial component of long-term prevention, particularly when it focuses on preventing recurrence of a condition.

In mental health and addiction treatment, a client may manage their symptoms or maintain sobriety, but clinical work is needed to focus on preventing relapse. In the criminal justice system, individuals convicted of a criminal offense may reoffend—an occurrence commonly referred to as "recidivism." In the field of homeless services, research, and policy, researchers, advocates, and other stakeholders have long been interested in "recidivism," "relapse," or "return" to homelessness, but this phenomenon has not been explicitly addressed in past federal policy responses. This dynamic has shifted in the United States in recent years. For example, the US Interagency Council on Homelessness—the federal entity with primary responsibility for efforts to address homelessness—has stated its desire to make homelessness "a rare, brief and one-time experience," thus implicitly articulating a goal of preventing repeated episodes of homelessness.[1]

Moreover, the US Department of Housing and Urban Development (HUD) now requires communities to track returns to homelessness as part of HUD's System Performance Measure no. 2 and considers performance on this measure in decisions about how federal homeless assistance dollars are allocated.[2] Similarly, the Department of Veterans Affairs (VA) has annually reported on returns to homelessness among veterans receiving services from the Supportive Services for Veteran Families program, its nationwide homelessness prevention and rapid rehousing program.[3] In this article, we focus on HUD and VA, which operate the two largest US homeless service systems, but we acknowledge that the topic applies to other homeless service systems domestically and internationally.

The increasing focus on returns to homelessness is a positive development given that a considerable proportion of individuals experiencing homelessness who successfully move to permanent housing experience homelessness again after some time (so "permanent" housing is aspirational). This is important to the field because repeated homelessness can lead, by definition, to chronic homelessness, which is associated with an array of adverse health and social consequences for individuals and can necessitate resource-intensive interventions.[4]

Yet, several key issues require greater consideration to employ and operationalize the concept of returning to homelessness for effective policy and program efforts to prevent repeated experiences of homelessness. Broadly speaking, these issues fall under two overarching questions: Over what time horizon should returns to homelessness be measured? What should count as a return to homelessness? In the remainder of this article, we engage with each of these questions with the ultimate aim of helping ensure that returns to homelessness are defined and measured in a way that makes them useful for driving improvements in the performance of homeless assistance systems. First, we draw on previous research as well as recent data from HUD and VA to provide context about the frequency and dynamics of returns to homelessness.

DATA ON RETURNS TO HOMELESSNESS

Researchers have taken interest in the phenomenon of returning to homelessness for several decades.[5–7] Studies conducted in the 1990s using administrative databases from emergency shelter systems in New York City and Philadelphia, Pennsylvania, found that returns to emergency shelter were common: more than 40% of men and more than a third of women who exited the single adult emergency shelter system in both cities reentered shelters within two years.[6] Related work found lower rates of returns to shelters for families.[7] A key finding from these studies was that risk of returns to homelessness was highest in the initial first few months immediately following the initial exit from a shelter, a finding corroborated in more recent research focused on rapid rehousing as well.[8]

More recent focus in the past two decades on returns to homelessness as measures of performance, such as that of HUD and VA, considers only those who exit the homeless service system to permanent housing—a group that earlier research found to face a lower risk of returns to shelter than those exiting to other destinations (e.g., transitional housing).[7] The focus solely on those who exit to permanent housing may reflect an assumption that those who leave the homeless service system to destinations other than permanent housing cannot be presumed to have definitively "exited" homelessness. Alternatively, the focus on those exiting to permanent housing may be appropriate for separating tertiary prevention cases from those who exit to destinations such as carceral facilities or hospitals. Moreover, many existing performance measures examine not just those exiting emergency shelter but also those who exit other programs to permanent housing, including those who exit from street outreach services, safe havens, and transitional housing programs.[2]

Available data suggest that most who exit one of these programs to permanent housing do not return to homelessness in the near term. For example, data from HUD System Performance Measure no. 2 track returns to homelessness at six months, one year, and two years.[9] In 2021, across 388 continuums of care (i.e., regional bodies that coordinate housing and services), the rate of returning to homelessness after exiting the homeless assistance system to a permanent housing destination was 9% within six months (range = 0%–35%), 13% within one year (range = 0%–39%), and 18% within two years (range = 0%–45%). In 2019 and 2020, the rates of returning to homelessness were highly similar at all follow-up periods.

The wide variability in return rates across continuums of care could be a function of a number of factors, including capacity and types of services available, the client populations served, documentation practices, and availability of staff and resources. VA data tell a similar story. In our analysis conducted across all VA homeless programs, we found that among veterans who exited to permanent housing destinations in fiscal year 2020, 5%, 9%, and 16% returned to homelessness at 6, 12, and 24 months, respectively. We defined a return as when a veteran returning to VA homeless programs was identified as experiencing homelessness at assessment for VA homeless services or upon entry into VA's rapid rehousing program.

Not only do rates of return vary by service area, but rates of return vary across program types, which is important to consider in performance monitoring. For example, HUD data indicate that the overall return rates at 6, 12, and 24 months among those exiting emergency shelters are 12%, 17%, and 22%, respectively, compared with 5%, 8%, and 12%, respectively, for those exiting permanent housing programs. Variation across program types may be attributable to differences in the populations served or the services provided by a particular program type. Although we value HUD's approach to tracking returns and consider it practical and useful, this variation underscores the point that, from an applied perspective, a refined approach to evaluating and using this measure may enhance the measure's effectiveness in driving performance improvement.

TIME HORIZON TO CAPTURE RETURNS

How long must an individual who formerly experienced homelessness be housed for the onset of a homeless episode to be considered a return to homelessness? At one extreme, if a long time horizon is employed, a person who experienced homelessness as a younger child but not again until decades later might be considered to have returned to homelessness. At the other extreme, if a short time horizon is employed, one could argue that a person who has an apartment leased in their name and then enters an emergency shelter after six months of stable housing is not returning to homelessness but experiencing a new, discrete episode of homelessness. Neither extreme approach is likely satisfactory.

HUD guidance on how to operationalize a return to homelessness uses a two-year time frame: it requires continuums of care to report on the proportion of individuals exiting homelessness to permanent housing who return within a period of up to 24 months from the date of their exit and counts individuals as "newly" experiencing homelessness if they have no record of entry into the homeless assistance system within the previous 24 months. There is not a concrete rationale of which we are aware for the use of this 24-month time frame, although it is consistent with the time frame used in early research examining returns to homelessness.[6,7] On the other hand, VA's Supportive Services for Veteran Families program tracks returns to homelessness for those who exit the rapid rehousing component of its program to permanent housing only for a follow-up of up to 12 months.[3]

HUD guidance indicates that its return to homelessness metric is intended to be used in conjunction with the number of persons newly experiencing homelessness who enter the system to assess the number of people experiencing homelessness in a given time frame. In this context, the time frame used to assess what is a return to homelessness versus a new episode has no effect on the number of people that a community identifies as experiencing homelessness. However, from the perspective of improving systems performance to reduce returns to homelessness, a more data-driven approach could yield more actionable information. For example, HUD guidance indicates that continuums of care should set targets for return rates that vary by program type.[10]

A potential extension of this guidance is to adjust follow-up times (e.g., three months, six months) according to how return rates vary by program type as baseline benchmarks for performance improvement. To be clear, HUD's guidance that communities track returns at 6-, 12-, and 24-month intervals is a straightforward and practical approach for setting targets. But an even more detailed program-specific approach could be useful. For example, if the majority of persons exiting a particular program who subsequently return do so within 6 months, the 12- and 24-month time points are less useful, and it may make sense to examine returns for that program at one-, three-, and six-month intervals instead. From a clinical practice and program improvement perspective, setting program-specific return time benchmarks could help inform critical periods after clients exit these programs in which it is especially important to bolster prevention efforts.

WHAT COUNTS AS A RETURN TO HOMELESSNESS

In considering measuring returns to homelessness, there are important data limitations to acknowledge and questions to answer about the types of homeless services that should be included and the duration of homelessness that qualifies as a return to homelessness.

Limitations

Current measures of returns to homelessness that HUD and VA use rely on administrative data from the homeless assistance system. However, homeless service systems will generally know a client has begun experiencing homelessness again only if they use a homeless service that is captured in the same data collection system. Therefore, a return to homeless services is an inexact proxy indicator for a return to homelessness because some individuals may begin to experience homelessness and not access homeless services. Depending on how broad of a definition of homelessness is used, other forms of housing instability (e.g., couch surfing) may be missed. In addition, individuals may begin to experience homelessness and access alternative service systems (e.g., residential substance use or mental health treatment) or have other touch points (e.g., domestic violence or religious shelters) that are not captured in centralized, linked data systems and thus may not be identified as experiencing homelessness.

If homeless service systems have the opportunity to integrate data sources from other service systems with their local Homeless Management Information System, it would likely yield a more comprehensive accounting of all client returns to homelessness. And to the extent possible, structured interviews and other corroborating data methods should be considered to validate samples of the data to ensure that data systems are being inclusive and accurate in capturing returns to homelessness. Doing so may also have clinical value by providing clients with a comprehensive safety net.

It may also be worth noting that the current performance measures capture returns to homelessness only after placement in permanent housing. Thus, they do not include individuals who exit a homeless assistance program before being placed in permanent housing (i.e., premature negative exits). Perhaps premature negative exits should be considered in a different category and tracked separately from returns to homelessness, but it may be important to recognize them as potential intervention points in clients' journeys in permanently exiting homelessness.

Types of Homeless Services That Count

Many communities offer a continuum of homeless programs ranging from brief housing assistance to permanent supported housing services. Thus, there is a question of whether a return to homelessness should be defined as a return to any homeless service or as including returns to only some broader or more narrow set of programs. For its part, HUD has operationalized a return to include only programs for which homelessness (per the statutory definition HUD uses) is an eligibility criterion.[11]

This is a reasonable approach, but including additional programs or tracking them separately may provide a more complete picture of how individuals who previously exited the homeless assistance system in a given community continue to use resources in that system. For example, use of homelessness prevention services does not typically require a person to experience homelessness, so including such services in a return measure would provide more information about the extent to which those who exit a system to permanent housing continue to rely on services provided by the system to remain stably housed. Similarly, including or separately tracking returns among those who complete intake for a community's coordinated entry system but are not literally homeless would also provide additional information about continued contacts of those who exited to permanent housing with the homeless assistance system. In both cases, such information would be useful for helping systems understand the scope of need for continued support for persons who have previously exited the system.

Length of Time Experiencing Homelessness

With some caveats, HUD guidance on returns to homelessness suggests that a person who spent one night in a shelter after exiting to permanent housing would be counted as having returned to homelessness. Again, this is practical to implement. But from a conceptual standpoint, it is reasonable to question the appropriateness of counting a person with a history of homelessness who spends only one night in a shelter as having returned to homelessness. This example may be extreme, but it does point to the fact that there is variation in what returning to homelessness means in terms of the longer-term trajectories of individuals' housing stability, and these differences have implications for interventions. Some may experience a return that is just a brief "blip" on an otherwise highly stable residential trajectory; others may experience a return episode of extended duration. From an intervention perspective, there is a big difference between these two types of return: the former may require little or no intervention, whereas the latter might be an indication of an individual in need of more intensive support.

Thus, at the systems level there may be great value in treating a return not simply as a yes or no indicator but by differentiating between different types of returns to determine the level of need in a functioning safety net. Doing so would provide more actionable information about the extent of need for intervention to assist those who have returned to homelessness to regain stable housing.

CONCLUSIONS

Helping individuals who exit homelessness remain stably housed and avoid repeated episodes of homelessness should be an important component of any strategic approach to end homelessness. Thus, understanding the extent to which this occurs has been of longstanding interest and has recently been incorporated into HUD and VA efforts to use data to drive system-level improvements. We agree with the logic in tracking returns and see the overall value of the approach HUD has adopted in tracking returns. However, additional considerations are needed of how this is defined and measured to be most useful to different homeless service systems.

We have highlighted some key decision points for possible refinements to this measure for programs and how they might be instructive for monitoring and improving system performance. We acknowledge that tracking returns to homelessness by different types and durations and using multiple data sources, as we suggest, will require data management resources and expertise. Having a metric that is too complicated or having too many metrics may also render them of limited utility. Nonetheless, we believe there is value in thinking more strategically about attending to returns to homelessness to support vulnerable populations, allocate resources, and have a clear understanding of causes of returns to homelessness. AJPH

CORRESPONDENCE

Correspondence should be sent to Jack Tsai, PhD, 1200 Pressler St, Houston, TX 77030 (e-mail: Jack.Tsai@uth.tmc.edu). Reprints can be ordered at http://www.ajph.org by clicking the "Reprints" link.

PUBLICATION INFORMATION

Full Citation: Tsai J, Byrne T. Returns to homelessness: key considerations for using this metric to improve system performance. *Am J Public Health*. 2023;113(5):490–494.

Acceptance Date: February 14, 2023.

DOI: https://doi.org/10.2105/AJPH.2023.307263

CONTRIBUTORS

J. Tsai conceptualized and wrote the article. T. Byrne helped write the article.

ACKNOWLEDGMENTS

J. Tsai's work on homelessness was supported by the National Institute on Minority Health and Health Disparities (grant 1R01MD018213-01). J. Tsai and T. Byrne are supported by the VA National Center on Homelessness Among Veterans.

Note. The views presented are of the authors alone and do not necessarily represent the US government or any federal agency.

CONFLICTS OF INTEREST

Neither author reports any conflicts of interest with this work.

REFERENCES

1. US Interagency Council on Homelessness. What does ending homelessness mean? June 4, 2018. Available at: https://www.usich.gov/all-in/goals/what-does-ending-homelessness-mean. Accessed August 25, 2022.
2. US Department of Housing and Urban Development. System performance measures: introductory guide. May 2015. Available at: https://www.hudexchange.info/resource/3894/system-performance-measures-introductory-guide. Accessed November 3, 2022.
3. US Department of Veterans Affairs. FY 2020 annual report. Supportive services for veteran families (SSVF). Available at: https://www.va.gov/homeless/ssvf/docs/ssvf_annual_report_fy20.pdf. Accessed February 28, 2023.
4. Tsai J, Mares AS, Rosenheck RA. A multi-site comparison of supported housing for chronically homeless adults: "housing first" versus "residential treatment first." *Psychol Serv.* 2010;7(4):219–232. https://doi.org/10.1037/a0020460
5. Dworsky AL, Piliavin I. Homeless spell exits and returns: substantive and methodological elaborations on recent studies. *Soc Serv Rev.* 2000;74(2):193–213. https://doi.org/10.1086/514476
6. Culhane DP, Kuhn R. Patterns and determinants of public shelter utilization among homeless adults in New York City and Philadelphia. *J Policy Anal Manage.* 1998;17(1):23–43. https://doi.org/10.1002/(SICI)1520-6688(199824)17:1<23::AID-PAM2>3.0.CO;2-J
7. Wong Y-LI, Culhane DP, Kuhn R. Predictors of exit and reentry among family shelter users in New York City. *Soc Serv Rev.* 1997;71(3):441–462. https://doi.org/10.1086/604265
8. Byrne T, Treglia D, Culhane DP, Kuhn J, Kane V. Predictors of homelessness among families and single adults after exit from homelessness prevention and rapid re-housing programs: evidence from the Department of Veterans Affairs Supportive Services for Veteran Families Program. *Hous Policy Debate.* 2016;26(1):252–275. https://doi.org/10.1080/10511482.2015.1060249
9. US Department of Housing and Urban Development. CoC system performance measures since FY 2015. May 2022. Available at: https://www.hudexchange.info/resource/5691/system-performance-measures-data-since-fy-2015. Accessed November 3, 2022.
10. US Department of Housing and Urban Development. Data quality and analysis for system performance improvement. July 2017. Available at: https://files.hudexchange.info/resources/documents/Data-Quality-and-Analysis-for-System-Performance-Improvement-Brief.pdf. Accessed November 3, 2022.
11. US Department of Housing and Urban Development. Four categories of the homeless definition. 2022. Available at: https://www.hudexchange.info/homelessness-assistance/coc-esg-virtual-binders/coc-esg-homeless-eligibility/four-categories. Accessed March 4, 2022.

Effectiveness of a Road Traffic Injury Prevention Intervention in Reducing Pedestrian Injuries, Barcelona, Spain, 2002–2019

Katherine Pérez, PhD, MPH, Elena Santamariña-Rubio, PhD, MPH, Josep Ferrando, MD, PhD, MPH, Maria José López, PhD, MPH, and Llorenç Badiella, MSC

This study aimed to evaluate the effectiveness of the Safe Routes to School (SRTS) intervention in Barcelona, Spain, at reducing the number of road traffic collisions and injuries in the school environment. It was a pre–post, quasi-experimental evaluation with a matched comparison group. Road traffic injuries were significantly reduced in the intervention schools—especially among school-age pedestrians—but not in the comparison schools. The SRTS program significantly improved road safety among children. (*Am J Public Health*. 2023;113(5):495–499. https://doi.org/10.2105/AJPH.2022.307216)

AJPH May 2023, Vol 113, No. 5

Many cities have promoted Safe Routes to School (SRTS) programs to make it easier for children to walk or cycle to school safely. Most studies have found that implementation of these programs increases active travel to school[1–3] and decreases road traffic injuries,[4–10] although there is controversy because of methodological limitations.[11]

INTERVENTION AND IMPLEMENTATION

Barcelona's SRTS program, called *Camí escolar, espai amic* (Safe route to school, friendly space), began with the aim of increasing children's and adolescents' personal autonomy, responsibility, and quality of life on their way to school or while walking around the neighborhood. The program promotes road safety education in schools through an educational program conducted within the school and the community, and through changes in the environment around the school.[12] After initial piloting, full deployment of SRTS began in 2006. Available data allowed us to evaluate a real-life policy with important public health implications. (For more details, see the Appendix, available as a supplement to the online version of this article at http://www.ajph.org).

PLACE, TIME, AND PERSONS

This is a pre–post, quasi-experimental evaluation study, with a matched comparison group. The intervention group was schools with the SRTS program, and the comparison group comprised schools without the SRTS program. The study area was defined as a buffer around the schools with a radius of about 200 meters (656 feet).

The inclusion and exclusion criteria were as follows: of the 152 schools with SRTS, we selected schools whose SRTS implementation year was after 2005 and whose inauguration year (street works and program implemented) was prior to 2016. All of the selected intervention schools had a pre- and postintervention period of at least four years per period; therefore, injury data include the years 2002 to 2019.

Inclusion and exclusion criteria for traffic collisions were as follows: we included traffic collisions with casualties occurring in the study area (buffer with a 200-m radius around the schools) from Monday to Friday from 7:00 AM to 9:30 AM, 12:00 PM to 3:00 PM, and 4:00 PM to 6:00 PM, from September 15 to June 23. Collisions occurring during Christmas and Easter holiday periods were excluded. (For more details, see the Appendix).

Outcome variables included the number of road traffic collisions involving casualties (total, children [defined as aged 0–16 years], and pedestrian children) and number of people injured (total, children, and pedestrian children).

Exposure variables included population in the area, available family income, and data on motor and active mobility and structure streets (for more detail, see Appendix).

To compare the results in the postintervention period versus the preintervention period, for each outcome measure, we fitted a generalized linear mixed model with Poisson distribution using the logarithm as a link function between expected values and explanatory variables. The explanatory variables included in the model were the group, the period (pre- vs postintervention), the interaction between group and period, and the year. To obtain a more precise fit, the model was also adjusted by the exposure variables.

PURPOSE

This study aimed to evaluate the effectiveness of the SRTS program carried out in Barcelona between 2006 and 2016 in reducing the number of road traffic collisions and injuries in the school environment.

EVALUATION AND ADVERSE EFFECTS

The study included 64 schools with SRTS programs implemented between 2006 and 2016, and 63 comparison schools, reaching 49 092 students in 2018 (intervention and comparison schools). A total of 15.0% of the schools were preschools (students aged 0–3 years), 55.1% were primary schools (students aged 4–11 years), and 29.9% were secondary schools (students aged 12–18 years). The proportion of public schools was higher in intervention than in comparison schools (75% and 60.3%, respectively), but there were no significant differences in the mean number of students per school: 367.8 (95% confidence interval [CI] = 306.7, 428.9) and 405.6 (95% CI = 320.2, 491.0), respectively.

The environmental characteristics of the intervention and comparison schools were similar. Differences were only found in the mean neighborhood income in 2017 and in the concentration of injured pedestrians in the school neighborhood in 2018. Available family income in the intervention school neighborhoods was significatively higher than in the comparison school neighborhoods (relative index = 112.1 and 99.8, respectively). The number of injured pedestrians per 100 meters of street was significatively lower for intervention schools (7.8) than for comparison schools (10.1).

In the intervention schools overall (aggregated), the total number of people injured was 2994 (annual mean = 272.2) in the preintervention period and 2284 (annual mean = 228.4) in the postintervention period. In the comparison schools, this number was 4061 (annual mean = 369.2) and 3196 (annual mean = 319.6), respectively (Table 1).

Per school, in the preintervention period, the annual mean number of injury road traffic collisions involving children and pedestrian children was significantly higher in the comparison schools than in the intervention schools. There were no differences in the annual school mean number of collisions involving children and pedestrian children (Table 1). In the postintervention period, the pattern was the same, although in general the annual school means were lower than in the preintervention period in both the intervention and comparison schools.

When we compared the results of the pre- and postintervention periods, the final adjusted models showed a significant reduction in the risk of collisions and people injured in the intervention schools, with a reduction of 11.7% in the number of injury collisions, 41.1% in the number of injury collisions involving children, and 43.3% in the number of injury collisions involving children pedestrians. For people injured, there was a reduction of 9.1% in the total injured, 36.6% in the number of children injured, and 39.9% in the number of children pedestrians injured (Table 2).

Among the comparison schools, there were no significant changes in outcomes between the pre- and postintervention periods (Table 2).

The significant difference in percentage change in the post- versus the preintervention period between intervention and comparison schools (significance of the interaction between intervention group and period) showed that the reduction in the intervention schools in the number of injury collisions involving children and pedestrian children could be attributable to the implementation of the SRTS program (Table 2).

SUSTAINABILITY

The SRTS program is currently beginning a new phase, with a greater focus on increasing safety in front of the school (*protegim les escoles*: we protect the schools).

PUBLIC HEALTH SIGNIFICANCE

The SRTS program, carried out in Barcelona between 2006 and 2016, showed a significant reduction in injuries in the intervention schools, which

TABLE 1— Injury Traffic Collisions and People Injured in Areas Surrounding Schools With an SRTS Program (200-Meter Buffer) and in Areas Surrounding Comparison Schools, by Intervention Period: Barcelona, 2002–2019

	Intervention Schools (n = 64)				Comparison Group Schools (n = 63)				
	All Schools Total	All Schools Annual Mean (95% CI)	Per School Range	Per School Annual Mean (95% CI)	All Schools Total	All Schools Annual Mean (95% CI)	Per School Range	Per School Annual Mean (95% CI)	Per School P^a (Intervention/ Comparison)
No. of road traffic collisions with injuries									
Preintervention	2994	272.2 (180.3, 364.1)	0–28	6.0 (5.6, 6.5)	4061	369.2 (249.1, 489.2)	0–37	8.2 (7.5, 8.9)	.001
Postintervention	2284	228.4 (119.9, 336.9)	0–28	5.7 (5.2, 6.2)	3196	319.6 (168.8, 470.4)	0–50	8.2 (7.3, 9.0)	.002
No. of collisions involving any injured person aged 0–16 y									
Preintervention	240	21.8 (13.2, 30.5)	0–4	0.5 (0.4, 0.5)	262	23.8 (14.5, 33.1)	0–4	0.6 (0.5, 0.6)	.033
Postintervention	120	12 (6.6, 17.4)	0–4	0.3 (0.2, 0.4)	169	16.9 (8.9, 24.9)	0–6	0.4 (0.4, 0.5)	.022
No. of collisions involving any injured pedestrians aged 0–16 y									
Preintervention	135	12.3 (6.8, 17.7)	0–3	0.3 (0.2, 0.3)	124	11.3 (6.7, 15.8)	0–3	0.3 (0.2, 0.3)	.76
Postintervention	66	6.6 (2.8, 10.4)	0–3	0.2 (0.1, 0.2)	97	9.7 (4.7, 14.7)	0–4	0.2 (0.2, 0.3)	.053
No. of people injured									
Preintervention	3478	316.2 (207.2, 425.2)	0–34	7 (6.4, 7.6)	4774	434 (292.4, 575.6)	0–47	9.6 (8.8, 10.5)	.001
Postintervention	2715	271.5 (141.7, 401.3)	0–33	6.8 (6.2, 7.4)	3720	372 (199.8, 544.2)	0–58	9.5 (8.5, 10.5)	.005
No. of injured persons aged 0–16 y									
Preintervention	251	22.8 (13.6, 32.1)	0–4	0.5 (0.4, 0.6)	288	26.2 (15.5, 36.8)	0–6	0.6 (0.5, 0.7)	.02
Postintervention	131	13.1 (7.1, 19.1)	0–4	0.3 (0.3, 0.4)	177	17.7 (9.2, 26.2)	0–6	0.5 (0.4, 0.5)	.024
No. of injured pedestrians aged 0–16 y									
Preintervention	136	12.4 (6.8, 17.9)	0–3	0.3 (0.2, 0.3)	131	11.9 (7.0, 16.8)	0–4	0.3 (0.2, 0.3)	.74
Postintervention	70	7 (3.0, 11.0)	0–3	0.2 (0.1, 0.2)	98	9.8 (4.7, 14.9)	0–4	0.3 (0.2, 0.3)	.06

Note. SRTS = Safe Routes to School.

[a]Significance of the nonparametric Wilcoxon rank-sum test (Mann-Whitney).

TABLE 2— Mean Number of Adjusted Annual Injury Collisions and Injured People, Adjusted Relative Risk, and Pre–Post Percentage Change in Surrounding Areas of Intervention and Comparison Schools: Barcelona, 2002–2019

	Intervention Schools (n = 64)				Comparison Group Schools (n = 63)				
	Adjusted Annual Mean Per School	SE	RR (95% CI)	Post/Pre % Change (95% CI)	Adjusted Annual Mean Per School	SE	RR (95% CI)	Post/Pre % Change (95% CI)	P[a]
No. of road traffic collisions with injuries									.14
Preintervention	4.72	0.34	1 (Ref)	1 (Ref)	5.03	0.36	1 (Ref)	1 (Ref)	
Postintervention	4.16	0.30	0.88 (0.80, 0.97)	−11.7 (−19.9, −2.7)	4.83	0.35	0.96 (0.88, 1.05)	−4.1 (−12.3, 5.0)	
No. of collisions involving injured persons aged 0–16 y									.019
Preintervention	0.43	0.04	1 (Ref)	1 (Ref)	0.44	0.04	1 (Ref)	1 (Ref)	
Postintervention	0.25	0.03	0.59 (0.47, 0.73)	−41.1 (−52.6, −27.0)	0.37	0.03	0.84 (0.68, 1.03)	−16.5 (−32.3, 3.1)	
No. of collisions involving injured pedestrians aged 0–16 y									.003
Preintervention	0.20	0.03	1 (Ref)	1 (Ref)	0.19	0.02	1 (Ref)	1 (Ref)	
Postintervention	0.12	0.02	0.57 (0.42, 0.77)	−43.3 (−58.3, −22.7)	0.20	0.03	1.05 (0.79, 1.38)	4.5 (−21.2, 38.5)	
No. of people injured									.87
Preintervention	5.44	0.39	1 (Ref)	1 (Ref)	6.14	0.44	1 (Ref)	1 (Ref)	
Postintervention	4.94	0.36	0.91 (0.82, 1.00)	−9.1 (−17.7, 0.4)	5.63	0.41	0.92 (0.84, 1.01)	−8.2 (−16.5, 0.9)	
No. of injured persons aged 0–16 y									.1
Preintervention	0.43	0.04	1 (Ref)	1 (Ref)	0.47	0.04	1 (Ref)	1 (Ref)	
Postintervention	0.28	0.03	0.63 (0.50, 0.81)	−36.6 (−50.4, −18.8)	0.39	0.04	0.82 (0.66, 1.03)	−17.8 (−34.3, 2.9)	
No. of injured pedestrians aged 0–16 y									.011
Preintervention	0.20	0.03	1 (Ref)	1 (Ref)	0.20	0.03	1 (Ref)	1 (Ref)	
Postintervention	0.12	0.02	0.60 (0.44, 0.82)	−39.9 (−55.9, −18.0)	0.20	0.03	1.00 (0.76, 1.34)	0.5 (−24.5, 33.6)	

Note. CI = confidence interval; RR = relative risk. Surrounding area defined as within a 200-meter buffer. Adjusted models include the explanatory variables, intervention group, period, the interaction between both terms and year, and the exposure variables, number of students of the school (log), number of inhabitants in the neighborhood (log), kilometers traveled by motor vehicles in the study area (log), and a quadratic term for the latter effect.

[a]Significance of the interaction between period and type of school (intervention, comparison), which allows us to assess whether the differences between intervention and comparison schools can be attributed to the intervention. It shows whether the difference pre–post in the intervention group is significantly different from the difference pre–post in the comparison group.

was not observed in the comparison schools. There was a notable decrease in the number of injured pedestrians, especially school-age pedestrians, which is the target population of the SRTS.

These results are relevant for two reasons. On the one hand, injuries were significantly reduced in the intervention schools but not in the comparison group, in the context of increasing road traffic injury rates in the city (although with decreasing severity). On the other hand, our results provide evidence of the effectiveness of the SRTS program in improving road safety and reducing road crashes and injuries, particularly among children, when there is controversy in the scientific literature.[9,11] Our study aimed to overcome the limitations reported in previous studies by using a quasi-experimental study, which controlled for major confounding factors through the study design and statistical analysis.

This study evaluates the health impacts of a policy developed outside the health sector. It provides evidence on how an infrastructure intervention contributes to health benefits, implementing health in all policies and reducing social inequities. AJPH

ABOUT THE AUTHORS

Katherine Pérez, Elena Santamariña-Rubio, Josep Ferrando, and Maria José López are with Agència de Salut Pública de Barcelona (ASPB), Barcelona, Spain. Katherine Pérez and Maria José López are also with CIBER Epidemiología y Salud Pública (CIBERESP), Institut d'Investigació Biomèdica Sant Pau (IIB SANT PAU), Barcelona, Spain. Llorenç Badiella is with Departament de Matemàtiques, Universitat Autònoma de Barcelona, Cerdanyola del Vallès, Barcelona, Spain.

CORRESPONDENCE

Correspondence should be sent to Katherine Pérez, Agència de Salut Pública de Barcelona (ASPB), Pl. Lesseps, 1, 08023 Barcelona, Spain (e-mail: cperez@aspb.cat). Reprints can be ordered at http://www.ajph.org by clicking the "Reprints" link.

PUBLICATION INFORMATION

Full Citation: Pérez K, Santamariña-Rubio E, Ferrando J, L Maria José, Badiella L. Effectiveness of a road traffic injury prevention intervention in reducing pedestrian injuries, Barcelona, Spain, 2002–2019. *Am J Public Health*. 2023;113(5): 495–499.

Acceptance Date: December 18, 2022.

DOI: https://doi.org/10.2105/AJPH.2022.307216

CONTRIBUTORS

K. Pérez and E. Santamariña designed and conceptualized the study. K. Pérez and J. Ferrando did the literature review. E. Santamariña and L. Badiella analyzed the data. All authors contributed to results and discussion. K. Pérez drafted the initial article, and all authors contributed to subsequent edits of the revised article.

ACKNOWLEDGMENTS

Llorenç Badiella received funding from the Spanish Ministry of Science, Innovation and Universities (grant RTI2018-096072-B-I00).

We thank Miquel Ruscalleda and Carme Ruiz (Road Safety and Mobility Program, Barcelona City Council); Pilar Lleonart, Gretel Vila, and Encarna Isanda (Municipal Institute of Education of Barcelona, IMEB); and Isaac Aparicio and Josep Clotet (Municipal Institute of Informatics, IMI).

CONFLICTS OF INTEREST

The authors have no conflicts of interest to declare.

HUMAN PARTICIPANT PROTECTION

The present article did not require institutional review board approval because we do not report human participant data.

REFERENCES

1. Chriqui JF, Taber DR, Slater SJ, Turner L, Lowrey KMG, Chaloupka FJ. The impact of state safe routes to school-related laws on active travel to school policies and practices in US elementary schools. *Health Place*. 2012;18(1):8–15. https://doi.org/10.1016/j.healthplace.2011.08.006
2. Hoelscher DM, Ganzar LA, Salvo D, et al. Effects of large-scale municipal safe routes to school infrastructure on student active travel and physical activity: design, methods, and baseline data of the Safe Travel Environment Evaluation in Texas Schools (STREETS) natural experiment. *Int J Environ Res Public Health*. 2022;19(3):1810. https://doi.org/10.3390/ijerph19031810
3. Stewart O, Moudon AV, Claybrooke C. Multistate evaluation of safe routes to school programs. *Am J Health Promot*. 2014;28(3 suppl):S89–S96. https://doi.org/10.4278/ajhp.130430-QUAN-210
4. DiMaggio C, Li G. Effectiveness of a safe routes to school program in preventing school-aged pedestrian injury. *Pediatrics*. 2013;131(2):290–296. https://doi.org/10.1542/peds.2012-2182
5. DiMaggio C, Brady J, Li G. Association of the Safe Routes to School program with school-age pedestrian and bicyclist injury risk in Texas. *Inj Epidemiol*. 2015;2(1):15. https://doi.org/10.1186/s40621-015-0038-3
6. DiMaggio C, Frangos S, Li G. National Safe Routes to School program and risk of school-age pedestrian and bicyclist injury. *Ann Epidemiol*. 2016; 26(6):412–417. https://doi.org/10.1016/j.annepidem.2016.04.002
7. Hagel BE, Macpherson A, Howard A, et al. The built environment and active transportation safety in children and youth: a study protocol. *BMC Public Health*. 2019;19(1):728. https://doi.org/10.1186/s12889-019-7024-6
8. Yu CY. How differences in roadways affect school travel safety. *J Am Plann Assoc*. 2015;81(3):203–220. https://doi.org/10.1080/01944363.2015.1080599
9. Lizarazo CG, Hall T, Tarko A. Impact of the Safe Routes to School Program: comparative analysis of infrastructure and noninfrastructure measures in Indiana. *J Transp Eng A Syst*. 2021;147(1). https://doi.org/10.1061/JTEPBS.0000480
10. Muennig PA, Epstein M, Li G, DiMaggio C. The cost-effectiveness of New York City's Safe Routes to School program. *Am J Public Health*. 2014; 104(7):1294–1299. https://doi.org/10.2105/AJPH.2014.301868
11. Kang B. Identifying street design elements associated with vehicle-to-pedestrian collision reduction at intersections in New York City. *Accid Anal Prev*. 2019;122:308–317. https://doi.org/10.1016/j.aap.2018.10.019
12. Saurí E, Sintes E, Truñó M. Avaluació Del Programa Camí Escolar, Espai Amic. 2017. Available at: https://institutinfancia.cat/es/mediateca/informe-davaluacio-programa-cami-escolar-espai-amic. Accessed August 7, 2022.

Engaging the Poultry Industry to Vaccinate Vulnerable Populations, Arkansas, 2021–2022

Austin Porter, DrPH, MPH, Pansy James, RN, and Cassie Cochran, MPH

See also Kapadia, p. 480.

The poultry and meatpacking industry is one of the largest in Arkansas and was associated with several COVID-19 outbreaks at the start of the pandemic. Marshallese and Hispanic workers account for much of the poultry and meatpacking workforce and were disproportionately affected. The Arkansas Department of Health held worksite vaccination clinics and administered 1794 doses. Of those doses, 1219 (67.9%) and 391 (21.8%) were administered to Hispanic and Marshallese workers, respectively. Vaccination efforts must target populations that have been disproportionately affected by the pandemic.
(*Am J Public Health*. 2023;113(5):500–503. https://doi.org/10.2105/AJPH.2023.307226)

AJPH May 2023, Vol 113, No. 5

According to the Poultry Federation, the state of Arkansas ranks third in the nation for poultry production, with more than 7.4 billion pounds of poultry produced in 2021.[1] Poultry production is the largest agriculture commodity in the state; with revenue of $5.1 billion, it accounts for approximately half of the state's total agriculture cash receipts.[1,2] Approximately 19 poultry and meatpacking companies are located in the state; employees are disproportionately Marshallese and Hispanic and may have limited access to health care.[3,4] Arkansas, with more than 15 000 Marshallese residents, has one of the largest Marshallese populations in the United States.[5] Marshall Islanders are free to migrate to the United States under a Compact of Free Association because the United States detonated more than 60 nuclear bombs that contaminated the Marshall Islands with radioactive pollution.[5,6]

During the Trump administration, an executive order was issued during the pandemic that declared the poultry and meatpacking industry to be critical infrastructure, which exempted the state from closing these plants.[7] In the early phase of the COVID-19 pandemic, employees of the poultry and meatpacking industry were among the first to experience notable outbreaks. Within six months of the pandemic, more than 3400 poultry and meatpacking employees in the state were infected with COVID-19.[3] Through fear of losing their jobs, poultry and meatpacking workers would often come to work while experiencing COVID-19–like symptoms, thus increasing the risk of spreading the virus to other workers and their family members.[3] Surveillance data showed that counties with poultry and meatpacking plants had higher rates of COVID-19 than counties without these plants.[8] Despite calls for a minimum two-week shutdown, poultry and meatpacking plants remained open in the state during the pandemic. Several plants made significant attempts to protect workers; these included the creation of health check-in stations and work station dividers, testing, leave time, and shifting of lines when necessary.

The Arkansas Department of Health (ADH) had worked with the poultry and meatpacking industry in previous years to offer worksite influenza and hepatitis A vaccines and tuberculosis tests for employees. When the COVID-19 vaccine became available, it was imperative to collaborate with poultry plants to vaccinate poultry and meatpacking workers at their workplace. The COVID-19 vaccine has been shown to significantly reduce the risk for severe illness that could result in hospitalization or death.[9]

INTERVENTION AND IMPLEMENTATION

To reach these workers, the ADH collaborated with any poultry and meatpacking facilities that would allow health department staff to come onsite to perform worksite vaccination clinics. The ADH established worksite vaccination clinics that provided not only the COVID-19 vaccine to employees, but also the influenza vaccine and educational material to those who were vaccine hesitant.

Vaccination providers were able to capture the race, ethnicity, and gender of those who were vaccinated at the worksite vaccination clinics. Additionally, the ADH employed Marshallese and Hispanic disease intervention specialists and community health workers who provided tailored educational material through pamphlets and visual media, made available in Spanish and Marshallese, to increase vaccination rates.

PLACE, TIME, AND PERSONS

Worksite vaccination efforts at poultry and meatpacking plants were initiated in the state starting in May 2021, shortly after the vaccine was available for food manufacturer workers. Employees would receive the vaccine while on break to avoid any disruption in plant productivity. Efforts to provide these clinics are ongoing. The worksite vaccination clinics were available to anyone, including eligible family members of employees. However, the target population was employees of poultry and meatpacking companies in the state.

PURPOSE

Worksite vaccination clinics were established by the ADH to assist state efforts in ensuring that employees of the poultry and meatpacking industry, who are disproportionately members of minority communities and hard-to-reach populations, had access to vaccinations, particularly the COVID-19 vaccine. The purpose of this evaluation was to describe these efforts to vaccinate this population in Arkansas.

EVALUATION AND ADVERSE EFFECTS

From May 2021 through April 2022, the ADH provided 30 worksite vaccination clinics located at 10 different poultry and meatpacking plant sites throughout the state (Table 1). Through these efforts, 1794 COVID-19 and 599 influenza vaccine doses were administered to industry employees and their family members. Among those, 1219 (67.9%) were Hispanic and 391 (21.8%) were Marshallese (Table 2). During August 2021 there were nine clinics held, at which nearly 750 doses of the COVID-19 vaccine were administered—the most in a one-month period. It was

TABLE 1— Number of COVID-19 and Influenza Vaccine Doses Administered at Poultry and Meatpacking Plants, by Time and Worksite Location: Arkansas, 2021–2022

Time of Worksite Vaccination Clinic	Company and Site	No. of COVID-19 Vaccine Doses Administered	No. of Influenza Vaccine Doses Administered
May 2021	Company A—Site 1	31	0
May 2021	Company B—Site 1	20	0
July 2021	Company C—Site 1	189	0
July 2021	Company C—Site 2	147	0
July 2021	Company A—Site 2	112	0
August 2021	Company A—Site 1	168	0
August 2021	Company A—Site 1	42	0
August 2021	Company A—Site 1	29	0
August 2021	Company D—Site 1	66	0
August 2021	Company A—Site 2	121	0
August 2021	Company A—Site 1	19	0
August 2021	Company C—Site 2	186	0
August 2021	Company A—Site 3	76	0
August 2021	Company A—Site 3	39	0
September 2021	Company D—Site 1	105	0
September 2021	Company D—Site 1	13	0
September 2021	Company D—Site 1	24	0
October 2021	Company D—Site 1	33	0
October 2021	Company C—Site 2	6	148
October 2021	Company C—Site 1	11	183
October 2021	Company C—Site 3	2	190
October 2021	Company C—Site 4	0	78
November 2021	Company D—Site 1	22	0
December 2021	Company D—Site 1	91	0
December 2021	Company D—Site 1	103	0
December 2021	Company D—Site 1	36	0
January 2022	Company D—Site 1	41	0
February 2022	Company D—Site 1	26	0
April 2022	Company B—Site 1	6	0
April 2022	Company E—Site 1	8	0

Note. Each row represents a separate clinic; there are 30 in total.

TABLE 2— Demographics of Patients Receiving COVID-19 Vaccine Doses at Poultry and Meatpacking Plants: Arkansas, 2021–2022

Demographic	No. (%) of Doses Administered (n = 1794)
Race	
Asian	143 (8.0)
Black	8 (0.4)
Marshallese	391 (21.8)
White	1252 (69.8)
Ethnicity	
Hispanic	1219 (67.9)
Non-Hispanic	575 (32.1)
Gender	
Female	777 (43.3)
Male	1017 (56.7)

difficult to estimate the reach of the intervention because demographic information on the total workforce was not provided to the program staff.

There were five companies that collaborated with the ADH in providing the clinics, with three companies accounting for more than 98% of the COVID-19 vaccine administered to employees and family members. There were 637 COVID-19 vaccine doses administered at Company A, the largest number administered among the five companies. The companies were committed to this effort and provided financial and other incentives for vaccinated employees, such as paid time off.

In addition to ADH staff on hand to answer questions, educational material was distributed to employees in an effort to address vaccine hesitancy. The ADH produced more than 30 promotional videos for the COVID-19 vaccine featuring trusted leaders and members of the community, of which 11 were in Spanish and two were in Marshallese. The ADH partnered with the Arkansas Coalition of Marshallese, the Marshallese Task Force, and the Marshallese Consul General to create videos and educational instruction. The ADH was not made aware of any adverse events.

SUSTAINABILITY

The ADH is committed to working with the poultry and meatpacking industry to address current and future public health issues by providing staff resources and time to conduct more worksite clinics. Given the success of this initiative, the industry may be willing to commit resources in the form of grants to sustain and expand these efforts to address other public health threats and emergencies.

Additionally, there are federal grant opportunities available to promote vaccination among vulnerable and hard-to-reach populations. The ADH intends to apply for these grants, and use the funds to maintain a workforce of 16 employees who will be committed to worksite clinics.

PUBLIC HEALTH SIGNIFICANCE

This program highlights the efforts of the ADH and the poultry and meatpacking industry to ensure that the COVID-19 and influenza vaccines were made available to a critical workforce that is largely Hispanic and Marshallese. These populations were disproportionately affected by the COVID-19 pandemic, particularly early in the pandemic.[3] Having access to vaccines is critically important to the Marshallese population because many may not be eligible for federal benefits such as Medicare if work requirements are not met.[4] A survey conducted by Hamel et al. indicated that Hispanic respondents may be reluctant to be vaccinated through fear of having to show government-issued identification and documentation.[10] To address this barrier, the ADH did not require recipients to provide any such documentation.

In addition to making the vaccine available, public health practitioners should provide education to those who may be vaccine hesitant. Many racial and ethnic minority groups, particularly Hispanics and African Americans, have shown greater rates of vaccine hesitancy than Whites.[11] The ADH employed a multipronged approach to reach minority and vulnerable populations. For example, to address COVID-19 vaccine disparities among the state's Black population, the ADH deployed health equity strike teams.[12] State and local departments of health aiming to increase vaccination rates among vulnerable populations employed by certain industries may consider this approach. AJPH

ABOUT THE AUTHORS

Austin Porter is with the Fay W. Boozman College of Public Health, University of Arkansas for Medical Sciences, and the Arkansas Department of Health, Little Rock. Pansy James and Cassie Cochran are with the Arkansas Department of Health.

Note. The views expressed in this article are solely those of the authors and do not necessarily represent the official views of the Arkansas Department of Health.

CORRESPONDENCE

Correspondence should be sent to Austin Porter, DrPH, MPH, 4301 W Markham Slot 820-12, Little Rock, AR 72205 (e-mail: aporter@uams.edu). Reprints can be ordered at http://www.ajph.org by clicking the "Reprints" link.

PUBLICATION INFORMATION

Full Citation: Porter A, James P, Cochran C. Engaging the poultry industry to vaccinate vulnerable populations, Arkansas, 2021–2022. *Am J Public Health*. 2023;113(5):500–503.

Acceptance Date: January 3, 2023.

DOI: https://doi.org/10.2105/AJPH.2023.307226

CONTRIBUTORS

A. Porter drafted the article and analyzed the data. P. James and C. Cochran provided significant revisions. P. James and C. Cochran conceptualized and coordinated the intervention.

CONFLICTS OF INTEREST

The authors have no conflicts of interest to disclose.

HUMAN PARTICIPANT PROTECTION

The institutional review board of the University of Arkansas for Medical Sciences designated this study as non–human participant research.

REFERENCES

1. The Poultry Federation. Industry facts & figures. Available at: https://www.thepoultryfederation.com/resources/facts-figures. Accessed December 12, 2022.
2. Division of Agriculture, University of Arkansas. YEAREND: Arkansas poultry stays strong. Division of Agriculture works to keep it that way with sustainability and animal well-being initiatives. Available at: https://aaes.uada.edu/news/poultry-yearender. Accessed August 29, 2022.
3. Center KE, Da Silva J, Hernandez AL, et al. Multidisciplinary community-based investigation of a COVID-19 outbreak among Marshallese and Hispanic/Latino Communities—Benton and Washington Counties, Arkansas, March–June 2020. *MMWR Morb Mortal Wkly Rep.* 2020;69(48):1807–1811. https://doi.org/10.15585/mmwr.mm6948a2
4. Kellams L. Marshallese families and the Affordable Care Act. Arkansas Advocates for Children and Families. November 2013. Available at: https://www.aradvocates.org/wp-content/uploads/Marshallese-Families-and-the-Affordable-Care-Act.pdf. Accessed December 12, 2022.
5. Marshallese Educational Initiative. Marshallese Community in Arkansas. Available at: https://www.mei.ngo/marshallese-in-arkansas. Accessed September 12, 2022.
6. Morris K. Navigating the Compact of Free Association: three decades of supervised self-governance. *U Haw L Rev.* 2018;41:384.
7. Herstein JJ, Degarege A, Stover D, et al. Characteristics of SARS-CoV-2 transmission among meat processing workers in Nebraska, USA, and effectiveness of risk mitigation measures. *Emerg Infect Dis.* 2021;27(4):1032–1038. https://doi.org/10.3201/eid2704.204800
8. Saitone TL, Aleks Schaefer K, Scheitrum DP. COVID-19 morbidity and mortality in US meatpacking counties. *Food Policy.* 2021;101:102072. https://doi.org/10.1016/j.foodpol.2021.102072
9. Moghadas SM, Vilches TN, Zhang K, et al. The impact of vaccination on coronavirus disease 2019 (COVID-19) outbreaks in the United States. *Clin Infect Dis.* 2021;73(12):2257–2264. https://doi.org/10.1093/cid/ciab079
10. Hamel L, Artiga S, Safarpour A, Stokes M, Brodie M. KFF COVID-19 Vaccine Monitor: COVID-19 vaccine access, information, and experiences among Hispanic Adults in the US. Kaiser Family Foundation. 2021. Available at: https://www.kff.org/coronavirus-covid-19/poll-finding/kff-covid-19-vaccine-monitor-access-information-experiences-hispanic-adults. Accessed December 12, 2022.
11. Nguyen LH, Joshi AD, Drew DA, et al. Racial and ethnic differences in COVID-19 vaccine hesitancy and uptake. *medRxiv.* Published online February 28, 2021. https://doi.org/10.1101/2021.02.25.21252402
12. Porter A, Wells S, Smith C, Zohoori N, Pro G, Smith MR. Deployment of health equity strike teams to address COVID-19 vaccine disparities in Arkansas, 2021. *Am J Public Health.* 2022;112(1):29–33. https://doi.org/10.2105/AJPH.2021.306564

Mpox Vaccine Interest Survey Prioritization and Data Flow: Maricopa County, Arizona, July–August 2022

Brandon J. Howard, MPH, Jennifer E. Collins, MPH, R. Nicholas Staab, MD, MSPH, Sonia Singh, Erika Lara, Melissa Kretschmer, CVT, MA, Lori Rehder, RN, BSN, Anne Dellos, Jessica R. White, DrPH, MS, and Ariella P. Dale, PhD, MPH

With increasing mpox cases in Maricopa County, Arizona, the county's health department launched a survey on July 11, 2022, to gather eligibility and contact data and provide clinic information to those interested in JYNNEOS as postexposure prophylaxis (PEP) or expanded postexposure prophylaxis (PEP++). Survey data were matched to case and vaccination data. Overall, 343 of the 513 respondents (66.9%) who reported close contact with an mpox case patient received PEP and 1712 of the 3379 respondents (50.7%) who were unsure of their contact status received PEP++. This outreach intervention connected potential close contacts unknown to MCDPH with PEP or PEP++. (*Am J Public Health*. 2023;113(5):504–508. https://doi.org/10.2105/AJPH.2023.307224)

AJPH May 2023, Vol 113, No. 5

The US mpox outbreak began on May 17, 2022, and was declared a public health emergency on August 4.[1,2] Response efforts broadened to include testing, treatment, and vaccination with JYNNEOS for postexposure prophylaxis (PEP) and expanded postexposure prophylaxis (PEP++).[3] The Centers for Disease Control and Prevention recommended prioritizing the two-dose JYNNEOS mpox vaccine for those with known exposure (PEP) or those with presumed exposure (PEP++) because of "certain risk factors and recent experiences that might make them more likely to have been recently exposed to mpox."[3] For our intervention, individuals at elevated risk of being exposed to mpox were defined as those who identify as men, nonbinary, or trans women and who have had intimate or sexual contact with men in a social or sexual venue, have had multiple or anonymous sexual partners of any gender identity, or give or receive money or other goods or services in exchange for sex with individuals of any gender identity.[4]

On June 9, 2022, a Maricopa County resident was confirmed as having the first case of mpox in Arizona.[5] Multiple mpox case patients reported numerous potential exposures, including anonymous sexual encounters, at a private event on July 2 with an estimated attendance of more than 500. As a result of limited vaccine supplies, difficulty reaching anonymous or unnamed individuals who had been exposed, and the 14-day window for PEP or PEP++, the Maricopa County Department of Public Health (MCDPH) rapidly developed and launched a vaccine interest survey on July 11 to assess PEP or PEP++ eligibility among the community at risk and disseminate vaccine information.

INTERVENTION AND IMPLEMENTATION

Permanent and temporary residents of Maricopa County enrolled in the online vaccine interest survey to receive information about mpox vaccine availability. The brief survey (which included eight questions) was distributed to attendees of private events with reported mpox exposures and named close contacts of patients with confirmed or probable mpox cases,[6] shared on the MCDPH Web site, and disseminated through community partners relevant to individuals at risk. Community partners tailored outreach and supported local vaccination events. Each individual provided their name, e-mail address, telephone number, and home zip code; attested whether they were an adult and currently residing or temporarily living in Arizona; and indicated whether they had had skin-to-skin contact or shared personal items with a person diagnosed with mpox and provided their most recent exposure date (if relevant).

After survey completion, all respondents immediately received an automated e-mail from MCDPH with current information on vaccine eligibility and upcoming vaccine events. Respondents then received weekly e-mail or text updates from MCDPH. Contact information for individuals who indicated that they had had skin-to-skin contact or shared personal items with a person diagnosed with mpox, regardless of the date of the most recent exposure, was sent to the MCDPH call center for PEP scheduling within one business day. Individuals attested to meeting PEP++ criteria at vaccination events. As vaccine supplies increased, the survey evolved from gathering data on eligibility for and interest in PEP to providing information to individuals on vaccine availability and events offering PEP++.

Survey responses were matched with vaccination data from the Arizona State Immunization Information System and data on mpox cases and potentially exposed individuals from the Arizona Medical Electronic Disease Surveillance Intelligence System. Vaccination frequencies were calculated among those who completed the vaccine interest survey, stratified by self-reported exposure type and whether individuals were identified as close contacts during case investigation. As vaccine supplies increased, scheduling a second dose to bolster protection became feasible. Matched data combined numerous sources of contact information, increasing the likelihood of reaching and scheduling those eligible for second doses.

PLACE, TIME, AND PERSONS

The intervention began after notification to MCDPH of a large event involving multiple mpox cases and quickly evolved to meet growing outbreak response needs as JYNNEOS vaccine availability increased. The intervention prioritized JYNNEOS for individuals with self-reported exposure to an mpox case patient (regardless of date of most recent exposure) who attested to residing in Maricopa County or the three neighboring counties of Gila, La Paz, and Pinal. Individuals provided information based on their current exposure status and were instructed to submit an additional response if their exposure status changed.

We shared the contact information of nonresident survey respondents with their home jurisdictions. We restricted our analysis to temporary and permanent residents of Maricopa County owing to the accessibility of close contact and vaccination data.

PURPOSE

As a result of increasing JYNNEOS vaccine availability[2] and the increased number of mpox cases, particularly among individuals with unnamed or anonymous contacts, there was an acute need for coordinated outreach to close contacts lacking contact information and to high-risk individuals interested in PEP++. MCDPH proactively collected contact information for individuals interested in PEP++ before vaccine supplies increased while prioritizing those with known exposure for prompt PEP scheduling. JYNNEOS should be administered as close to the exposure date as possible (within four days to prevent the onset of clinical disease and within 14 days to attenuate symptoms but potentially not prevent clinical disease altogether).[7] As vaccine availability allowed, JYNNEOS doses allocated to Maricopa County that were not needed for PEP were used as PEP++ at community events for those who self-reported meeting the high-risk criteria.[3]

EVALUATION AND ADVERSE EFFECTS

From July 11 to August 31, 2022, 10 226 responses were received for Maricopa County residents representing 8708 unique individuals who completed the survey and regularly received sharable updates on vaccine availability and events (Table 1). As of September 1, 3819 (43.9%) respondents had received at least one dose of JYNNEOS as PEP or PEP++; 343 (9.0%) were prioritized for immediate PEP scheduling owing to reported exposure (Table 1). A sensitivity analysis comparing individual responses and unique respondents yielded similar proportions. Respondents eligible for PEP received their first dose of JYNNEOS within a median of four days (interquartile range [IQR] = 4) of survey submission and PEP++ within eight days (IQR = 9); this was influenced by vaccine supply and next available MCDPH vaccine event. We identified an additional 3116 vaccinated individuals using data from the Arizona State Immunization Information System who did not complete the survey or were unmatched as a result of collection of limited demographic information (Table 2).

Of the 6935 individuals vaccinated with at least one dose of JYNNEOS as of September 1, 3819 (55.1%) completed the vaccine interest survey (Table 2). Most individuals who received at least one dose of JYNNEOS identified as

TABLE 1— Vaccine Received Among Vaccine Interest Survey Respondents, by Reported Exposure: Maricopa County, AZ, July 11–August 31, 2022

	No. (%)				
Vaccine Status	**Total Unique Respondents[a] (n = 8708)**	**Total Reporting Exposure (n = 513)**	**Total Unsure of Exposure Status (n = 3379)**	**Total Reporting No Known Exposure (n = 4816)**	**Total Matched to Named Close Contacts[b] During Case Investigation (n = 75[c])**
Received vaccine	3819 (43.9)	343 (66.9)	1712 (50.7)	1764 (36.6)	45 (60.0)
Did not receive vaccine	4889 (56.1)	170 (33.1)	1667 (49.3)	3052 (63.4)	30 (40.0)

Note. Data include all submissions from July 11 to August 31, 2022, and vaccinations provided on or before September 1, 2022, to allow for individuals to be scheduled for vaccination. The vaccination record data cutoff was October 31, 2022, to allow for data entry. Survey respondents were included in the analysis if they provided at least one form of contact information (telephone or e-mail) and their first and last names for matching to vaccine records.

[a]The most recent submission was used for 1220 individuals who responded more than once.
[b]Named close contacts were identified by people with mpox during standard case investigation per the Centers for Disease Control and Prevention definition.
[c]Of the 75 close contacts identified during case investigation between July 11 and August 31, 2022, who were matched to a survey respondent, 24 (32%) were referred for postexposure prophylaxis and 51 (68%) were eligible for expanded postexposure prophylaxis.

TABLE 2— Demographic Characteristics of Maricopa County, AZ, Residents Vaccinated With JYNNEOS Mpox Vaccine by Participation in Vaccine Interest Survey, July 11–September 1, 2022

	Median (Min–Max) or No. (%)			
Characteristic	**All Individuals Vaccinated With at Least One Dose (n = 6935)**	**Vaccinated Individuals Who Completed the Vaccine Interest Survey[a] (n = 3819)**	**Vaccinated Individuals Who Did Not Complete the Vaccine Interest Survey (n = 3116)**	***P*[b]**
Age,[c] y	38 (14–99)	38 (14–99)	37 (15–84)	
Age group				> .99
< 18 years	3 (< 0.1)	2 (0.1)	1 (< 0.1)	
≥ 18 years	6932 (> 99.9)	3817 (99.9)	3115 (> 99.9)	
Race[d]				< .01
American Indian or Alaska Native[e]	277 (4.0)	132 (3.5)	145 (4.7)	
Asian or Pacific Islander	296 (4.3)	161 (4.2)	135 (4.3)	
Black or African American	377 (5.4)	217 (5.7)	160 (5.1)	
White	4370 (63.0)	2535 (66.4)	1835 (58.9)	
Other	801 (11.6)	415 (10.9)	386 (12.4)	
Unknown	814 (11.7)	359 (9.4)	455 (14.6)	
Hispanic or Latino ethnicity[f]				< .01
Hispanic or Latino	1611 (23.2)	892 (23.4)	719 (23.1)	
Not Hispanic or Latino	3918 (56.5)	2278 (59.6)	1640 (52.6)	
Unknown	1406 (20.3)	649 (17.0)	757 (24.3)	

Note. Data include all submissions from July 11 to August 31, 2022, and vaccinations provided on or before September 1, 2022, to allow for individuals to be scheduled for vaccination. The vaccination record data cutoff was October 31, 2022, to allow for data entry.

[a]Individuals who completed the vaccine interest survey more than once are represented only once.
[b]The Fisher exact test was used to assess differences between age groups; the χ^2 test was used for race and ethnicity.
[c]Age at administration of first dose of JYNNEOS.
[d]Race was self-reported according to the mutually exclusive categories listed.
[e]Vaccine records were geocoded to determine the appropriate jurisdiction. If a vaccine record was geocoded to a tribal jurisdiction, regardless of the physical county of residence, the record would not be present in Maricopa County vaccine data.
[f]Ethnicity was self-reported according to the mutually exclusive categories listed.

White (63.0%), adults (more than 99.9%), and non-Hispanic or Latino (56.5%; Table 2). Anecdotally, e-mail and text updates from MCDPH were reported by media outlets and were shared with others through social media, social networks, and distribution lists. We did not evaluate the extent of distribution by MCDPH or community partners or ask individuals receiving the vaccine how they learned of vaccination events.

Given sensitivities around this diagnosis, the affected community, and modes of transmission, the survey was designed to maintain privacy, not be overly burdensome on respondents, and collect only pertinent contact information and data on eligibility criteria. For example, age category was collected instead of date of birth. This limited our ability to match survey respondents to vaccine records. Numerous responses were incomplete (e.g., missing name) and could not be matched to vaccine or case/contact data but still received updates to an entered phone number or e-mail. MCDPH included the call center telephone number on its Web site, with support for non-English speakers, and in all outreach communications to decrease sign-up barriers for individuals with limited Internet access.

Of the 767 individuals identified as close contacts during case investigation between July 11 and August 31, 609 (79.4%) had information available for matching; 75 (12.3%) were matched to a survey response, of whom 45 (60.0%) received at least one dose of JYNNEOS. Of all close contacts reported, 632 (82.4%) were identified as health care workers during standard case investigation, highlighting the limited number of social or household contacts provided. Named social and household contacts were not evaluated outside of the survey; however, potentially exposed health care workers were first vetted by public health personnel to determine eligibility for PEP. Our process attempted to connect anonymous or unknown contacts and high-risk individuals with PEP or PEP++ while subverting the stigma associated with being named a close contact during a standard case investigation.

Potential adverse effects of the intervention included the possibility of delays in scheduling of mpox PEP if contact information was incorrect and unwanted viewing by others of text and e-mail communications mentioning mpox.

SUSTAINABILITY

As JYNNEOS becomes more available through local community vaccinators, this intervention will be adaptable and flexible with respect to keeping individuals informed about vaccine availability and events.

PUBLIC HEALTH SIGNIFICANCE

Vaccination is one of the most effective interventions to reduce the risk of contracting and spreading mpox.[3] Rapid outreach is critical to prevent the spread of mpox but faces challenges when potentially exposed individuals are not named. By quickly conducting outreach via a survey, MCDPH was able to connect individuals to PEP and PEP++ through regular communications regarding vaccination events that were also shared with others who did not directly engage with public health. This adaptable intervention allows local public health departments to use limited resources to effectively prioritize vaccine distribution for interested individuals who are most at risk and minimize stigma. AJPH

ABOUT THE AUTHORS

The authors are with the Maricopa County Department of Public Health, Phoenix, AZ.

CORRESPONDENCE

Correspondence should be sent to Brandon J. Howard, MPH, 4041 N Central Ave, Suite 600, Phoenix, AZ 85012 (e-mail: brandon.howard@maricopa.gov). Reprints can be ordered at http://www.ajph.org by clicking the "Reprints" link.

PUBLICATION INFORMATION

Full Citation: Howard BJ, Collins JE, Staab RN, et al. Mpox vaccine interest survey prioritization and data flow: Maricopa County, Arizona, July–August 2022. *Am J Public Health*. 2023;113(5):504–508.

Acceptance Date: January 3, 2023.

DOI: https://doi.org/10.2105/AJPH.2023.307224

CONTRIBUTORS

B. J. Howard was the lead author and performed the analysis under guidance from J. E. Collins, J. R. White, and A. P. Dale. A. P. Dale provided executive oversight for the analysis, writing, and editing. J. E. Collins, R. N. Staab, S. Singh, E. Lara, M. Kretschmer, L. Rehder, A. Dellos, and J. R. White provided additional editorial oversight. All of the authors were involved with intervention design and implementation and contributed significantly to the article and the work described.

ACKNOWLEDGMENTS

The outbreak response work associated with this article was partially funded by the Centers for Disease Control and Prevention Public Health Emergency Preparedness Cooperative Agreement.

We acknowledge community partners and organizations, Rebecca Sunenshine, the Maricopa County Department of Public Health (MCDPH) Mpox Response Incident Command, the MCDPH CARES Team, the MCDPH Clinical Services Division, Machrina Leach, Kelsey Andrews, Nicole M. Jarrett, James Matthews, Angela Moreth, Thomas Shows, Nicholas Moyte, Karen Zabel, and Katherine C. Hobbs.

CONFLICTS OF INTEREST

The authors have no conflicts of interest to disclose.

HUMAN PARTICIPANT PROTECTION

This article details routine public health practice, and all data are reported in aggregate in accordance with local, state, and federal policies.

REFERENCES

1. US Department of Health and Human Services. Determination that a public health emergency exists. Available at: https://aspr.hhs.gov:443/legal/PHE/Pages/monkeypox-4Aug22.aspx. Accessed August 17, 2022.
2. Philpott D, Hughes CM, Alroy KA, et al. Epidemiologic and clinical characteristics of monkeypox cases—United States, May 17–July 22, 2022. Available at: https://www.cdc.gov/mmwr/volumes/71/wr/mm7132e3.htm. Accessed August 30, 2022.
3. Centers for Disease Control and Prevention. Vaccination strategies. Available at: https://www.cdc.gov/poxvirus/monkeypox/interim-considerations/overview.html. Accessed August 30, 2022.
4. Centers for Disease Control and Prevention. Mpox vaccine basics. Available at: https://www.cdc.gov/poxvirus/monkeypox/vaccines/vaccine-basics.html. Accessed December 15, 2022.
5. Maricopa County Government. Maricopa County announces first probable monkeypox case. Available at: https://www.maricopa.gov/CivicAlerts.aspx?AID=2512. Accessed August 17, 2022.
6. Centers for Disease Control and Prevention. Case definitions for use in the 2022 mpox response. Available at: https://www.cdc.gov/poxvirus/monkeypox/clinicians/case-definition.html. Accessed September 8, 2022.
7. Centers for Disease Control and Prevention. Interim clinical considerations for use of JYNNEOS and ACAM2000 vaccines during the 2022 U.S. mpox outbreak. Available at: https://www.cdc.gov/poxvirus/monkeypox/clinicians/smallpox-vaccine.html. Accessed August 17, 2022.

Impact of a Large Healthy Start Program on Perinatal Outcomes, South Carolina, 2009–2019

Jihong Liu, ScD, Longgang Zhao, MS, MBBS, Xingpei Zhao, MS, MBBS, Eric Mishio Bawa, MPHIL, Kimberly Alston, MA, Sabrina Karim, PhD, Anwar T. Merchant, PhD, DMD, Jun Tang, PhD, and Sara Wilcox, PhD

Using linked birth and death certificates for participants served by a Healthy Start program in South Carolina and community controls, we found that the Healthy Start program contributed to significant improvements in prenatal care, breastfeeding initiation, and participation in the Special Supplemental Nutrition Program for Women, Infants, and Children and significant reductions in inadequate weight gain and large-for-gestational-age births. However, Healthy Start participants were more likely to gain excessive weight during pregnancy, and there were no significant differences in perinatal outcomes. (*Am J Public Health*. 2023;113(5):509–513. https://doi.org/10.2105/AJPH.2023.307232)

AJPH May 2023, Vol 113, No. 5

The federal Healthy Start (HS) program is one of the nation's earliest initiatives focusing on reducing infant mortality in high-risk communities where infant mortality rates are 1.5 to 2.5 times the national average.[1] Yet, this program has been categorized as one of the 31 early childhood home visit models that do not meet the criteria for an evidence-based service delivery model.[2]

Previous research has mostly evaluated the effects of the HS program on infant outcomes. Few studies have assessed its impact on health behaviors, public service use, and maternal outcomes. Researchers in several studies have used propensity score matching methods to make control and HS groups comparable with respect to sociodemographic and clinical risk factors.[3–7] However, these studies have included only small numbers of HS participants,[4–6] raising concerns about representativeness. Thus, there is an urgent need to conduct a population-based program evaluation involving rigorous methods, more recent data, larger sample sizes, and more outcome domains.

INTERVENTION AND IMPLEMENTATION

The Midlands Healthy Start (MHS) program, a federally funded HS program, has been serving residents in the Midlands region of South Carolina since 1998. The goals of MHS are to eliminate racial disparities in perinatal health by mainly serving low-income African American and Hispanic populations; improving the health of high-risk women and their infants; addressing gaps in screening, assessment, and referral for depression and other social needs among pregnant and postpartum women; increasing access to prenatal care; and removing barriers to health care access. MHS participants are enrolled during pregnancy and followed up to 18 months after delivery. The core intervention strategies include case management, outreach and recruitment, health education, a local health system action plan, and interconception care for high-risk women and infants. The case management intervention includes risk assessment, referral, monitoring, facilitation, and follow-up with respect to use of needed services.

PLACE, TIME, AND PERSONS

This retrospective cohort study included all MHS participants (n = 7203) who delivered a singleton live birth and lived in the South Carolina counties of Richland and Fairfield between June 2009 and August 2014 or Lexington and Sumter between January 2011 and January 2019. The control group included non-MHS women who delivered singleton live births in the respective counties during the study period (n = 48 826; Figure A of the Appendix, available as a supplement to the online version of this article at http://www.ajph.org). Linked birth and infant death certificate data were used.

PURPOSE

In this study, we evaluated the impact of the MHS program on prenatal care, public service use, and maternal and infant health outcomes.

EVALUATION AND ADVERSE EFFECTS

Compared with non-MHS controls, MHS participants were younger at childbirth (24.8 vs 27.9 years) and had a higher mean prepregnancy body mass index (28.7 vs 27.5). A majority of MHS participants were non-Hispanic African American (74.5%), whereas a majority of non-MHS controls were non-Hispanic White (60.2%). MHS participants were more likely to have a high school education or less (53.4% vs 29.4%), to be receiving Medicaid (79.9% vs 40.3%), and to have been obese before pregnancy (36.4% vs 29.0%). The percentage of women with adverse pregnancy histories was lower among those taking part in the MHS program (23.5% vs 25.2%; Table 1).

The incidence of adverse maternal and infant health and behavioral outcomes was significantly higher among MHS participants (Table 2 and Appendix Table A). As a result, we applied propensity score stratification to ensure that the control group met the criterion of baseline equivalency.[8] Generalized linear mixed models stratified by propensity score quintiles[9] were used to evaluate whether there were differences between MHS and non-MHS women in terms of the outcomes of interest.

In the pooled sample, MHS participants had 19% lower odds of having large-for-gestational-age babies than non-MHS controls (adjusted odds ratio [AOR] = 0.81; 95% confidence interval [CI] = 0.67, 0.99). MHS participants had higher odds of participating in the Special Supplemental Nutrition Program for Women, Infants, and Children (WIC; AOR = 2.68; 95% CI = 2.49, 2.89) and having initiated breastfeeding in the hospital (AOR = 1.14; 95% CI = 1.03, 1.26). There were no significant differences between MHS and non-MHS women with respect to other outcomes, specifically composite adverse birth outcomes, low birth weight, small-for-gestational-age babies, preterm births, infant death, smoking during pregnancy, diabetes or hypertension during pregnancy, and cesarean deliveries (Table 2).

We conducted sensitivity analyses using a propensity score adjustment approach and multivariable adjusted models (Table 2). The findings from these two approaches were similar, but other significant associations were revealed. Compared with non-MHS controls, MHS participants had 14% lower odds of having inadequate prenatal care (AOR = 0.86; 95% CI = 0.80, 0.92). Also, MHS participants had lower odds of gaining weight below the Institute of Medicine's recommended total weight gain during pregnancy (AOR = 0.90; 95% CI = 0.85, 0.96), but they had higher odds of gaining weight above the recommended gain (AOR = 1.10; 95% CI = 1.04, 1.16). County-specific models showed lower odds of low birth weight among MHS participants than among non-MHS controls in Lexington and Sumter counties and higher odds of adverse birth outcomes and infant mortality in Richland and Fairfield counties (Appendix Tables B and C).

SUSTAINABILITY

HS programs are sustainable because the federal HS initiative has been authorized through the Public Health Service Act and has been implemented in the United States since 1991.

PUBLIC HEALTH SIGNIFICANCE

The MHS program did not significantly reduce the risk of adverse birth outcomes such as low birth weight, preterm delivery, and infant mortality in a high-risk and underserved population. However, program participation was associated with significant reductions in inadequate prenatal care, large-for-gestational-age births, and inadequate weight gain during pregnancy. The HS program had a positive impact on participants in terms of breastfeeding practices and participation in other public service programs (e.g., WIC).

Life course theories emphasize the importance of intervening before pregnancy if risk factors are present.[10,11] A large proportion of participants initiated HS services in the second or third trimester, leaving little time for program impact on maternal and infant health outcomes among these high-risk women. Thus, strategies are needed on how to serve high-risk women early in pregnancy or preconceptionally. It would also be helpful to understand how use of specific services and duration of program involvement differentially relate to outcomes.

Furthermore, the MHS doubled the total number of women served in Richland and Fairfield counties over a five-year time window relative to the

TABLE 1— Comparison of MHS Participants and Community Controls According to Selected Sociodemographic, Behavioral, and Medical Characteristics: South Carolina, 2009–2019

Characteristic	Pooled Sample			Lexington and Sumter 2011–2019			Richland and Fairfield 2009–2014		
	Non-MHS (n = 48 826)	MHS (n = 7203)	Standardized Difference[a]	Non-MHS (n = 31 105)	MHS (n = 2067)	Standardized Difference[a]	Non-MHS (n = 17 721)	MHS (n = 5136)	Standardized Difference[a]
Mean maternal age, y	27.9	24.8	−0.55	27.6	25.3	−0.42	28.4	24.6	−0.67
Mean maternal prepregnancy BMI	27.5	28.7	0.15	27.8	29.2	0.17	27.1	28.5	0.19
Maternal age, y, %			0.56			0.42			0.68
< 20	6.5	17.2		6.6	16.4		6.2	17.4	
20–24	23.6	37.4		25.1	33.9		21.0	38.8	
25–29	30.8	25.6		31.5	26.9		29.6	25.0	
30–34	25.9	13.1		24.9	14.7		27.8	12.5	
≥ 35	13.2	6.7		11.9	8.0		15.4	6.2	
Maternal race/ethnicity, %			1.00			0.78			0.86
Non-Hispanic White	60.2	18.9		67.1	32.6		48.1	13.3	
Non-Hispanic African American	32.4	74.5		25.7	59.7		44.2	80.4	
Hispanic	4.2	5.7		4.4	6.4		3.9	5.5	
Non-Hispanic other	3.1	1.0		2.7	1.3		3.8	0.8	
Maternal education, %			0.65			0.61			0.87
< high school	9.6	22.4		10.5	21.8		8.0	22.6	
High school or equivalent	19.8	31.0		21.9	33.2		16.1	30.1	
Some college	36.7	36.8		38.0	35.5		34.4	37.4	
Bachelor's degree	21.0	7.0		19.0	6.8		24.5	7.0	
Graduate school	12.9	2.8		10.6	2.7		16.9	2.9	
Medicaid medical insurance, %	40.3	79.9	0.88	41.3	74.2	0.71	38.4	82.1	1.00
Nulliparous, %	41.7	49.2	0.15	40.6	46.8	0.13	43.7	50.1	0.13
Prepregnancy BMI category, %			0.20			0.19			0.23
Underweight (< 18.5 kg/m^2)	3.2	4.1		3.1	4.3		3.3	4.1	
Normal weight (18.5–24.9 kg/m^2)	39.1	33.6		37.0	31.4		42.8	34.5	
Overweight (25.0–29.9 kg/m^2)	24.9	24.5		23.9	21.5		26.6	25.7	
Obese (≥ 30.0 kg/m^2)	29.0	36.4		29.9	38.0		27.3	35.8	
Missing	3.9	1.4		6.1	4.9				
Smoking before pregnancy, %	12.4	15.8	0.10	13.4	14.2	0.03	10.9	16.4	0.16
Composite disease history score ≥ 1, %[b]	25.2	23.5	−0.04	25.7	24.5	−0.03	24.3	23.0	−0.03

Note. BMI = body mass index (defined as weight in kilograms divided by the square of height in meters); MHS = Midlands Healthy Start.

[a]Standardized differences are differences in means or percentages divided by standard errors. Absolute values above 0.20 indicate imbalances between groups.

[b]The presence of any of the following conditions: history of preterm birth, previous cesarean, prepregnancy diabetes, prepregnancy hypertension, and other previous poor pregnancy outcomes.

TABLE 2— Associations Between Healthy Start Program Participation and Health Outcomes in Four South Carolina Counties (Pooled Sample): 2009–2019

	Non-MHS, %	MHS, %	AOR (95% CI)		
			Propensity Score Stratification[a]	Propensity Score Adjustment[b]	Multivariable Adjusted Model[c]
Composite adverse birth outcome[d]	18.9	25.9	1.07 (0.99, 1.15)	0.98 (0.92, 1.05)	1.00 (0.94, 1.07)
Low birth weight (< 2500 g)	7.2	10.7	0.91 (0.78, 1.07)	0.96 (0.87, 1.05)	0.97 (0.89, 1.07)
Very low birth weight (< 1500 g)	1.2	1.8	0.99 (0.91, 1.08)	0.93 (0.75, 1.15)	0.92 (0.75, 1.13)
Small-for-gestational-age birth[e]	11.1	16.2	1.09 (0.94, 1.26)	0.97 (0.89, 1.05)	0.99 (0.92, 1.07)
Large-for-gestational-age birth[f]	10.5	6.2	0.81 (0.67, 0.99)	0.96 (0.86, 1.07)	0.93 (0.84, 1.04)
Preterm birth (< 37 weeks)	8.6	10.5	0.90 (0.69, 1.16)	0.96 (0.88, 1.06)	0.96 (0.88, 1.05)
Very preterm birth (< 32 weeks)	1.3	1.8	0.92 (0.82, 1.04)	0.87 (0.71, 1.08)	0.88 (0.72, 1.08)
Infant death	0.4	0.7	1.36 (0.75, 2.49)	1.40 (0.97, 2.03)	1.33 (0.93, 1.90)
Inadequate prenatal care[g]	17.0	23.2	1.12 (0.90, 1.40)	0.86 (0.80, 0.92)	0.87 (0.82, 0.93)
Smoking during pregnancy	9.1	12.0	1.11 (0.94, 1.30)	1.02 (0.93, 1.11)	1.19 (1.03, 1.38)
Gestational weight gain[h]					
Excessive	61.2	60.5	0.97 (0.84, 1.13)	1.10 (1.04, 1.16)	1.08 (1.02, 1.15)
Adequate	12.8	11.3	0.97 (0.83, 1.14)	0.96 (0.88, 1.05)	0.96 (0.88, 1.04)
Inadequate	21.6	26.3	1.06 (0.85, 1.33)	0.90 (0.85, 0.96)	0.93 (0.88, 0.99)
WIC participation	38.8	80.5	2.68 (2.49, 2.89)	2.52 (2.34, 2.71)	3.05 (2.84, 3.28)
Breastfeeding initiation at birth	75.1	64.3	1.14 (1.03, 1.26)	1.19 (1.12, 1.26)	1.13 (1.06, 1.20)
Diabetes during current pregnancy	6.4	7.1	1.01 (0.81, 1.25)	1.10 (0.98, 1.22)	1.17 (1.05, 1.31)
Hypertension during current pregnancy	6.2	6.5	1.04 (0.92, 1.18)	1.00 (0.90, 1.12)	0.99 (0.88, 1.10)
Primary cesarean section	19.4	20.7	1.09 (1.00, 1.18)	0.99 (0.92, 1.06)	1.00 (0.93, 1.07)
Low-risk cesarean section[i]	10.8	12.5	1.05 (0.96, 1.16)	1.02 (0.93, 1.11)	1.02 (0.96, 1.09)
Cesarean section	33.4	31.8	1.00 (0.97, 1.03)	0.96 (0.91, 1.02)	0.95 (0.89, 1.02)

Note. AOR = adjusted odds ratio; CI = confidence interval; MHS = Midlands Healthy Start; WIC = Special Supplemental Nutrition Program for Women, Infants, and Children.

[a]Propensity scores were created on the basis of maternal age, maternal education, maternal race/ethnicity, Medicaid health insurance, nulliparous status, prepregnancy body mass index category, smoking before pregnancy, composite disease history score, year of birth, and county of residence. AORs and 95% CIs were for MHS vs non-MHS participation from generalized linear mixed models considering multiple pregnancies over the study period and stratified by propensity score quintile.
[b]AORs and 95% CIs were for MHS vs non-MHS participation from generalized linear mixed models considering multiple pregnancies over the study period and adjusted for propensity score.
[c]AORs and 95% CIs were for MHS vs non-MHS participation from generalized linear mixed models considering multiple pregnancies over the study period and adjusted for all of the covariates listed in Table 1 along with year of birth and county of residence.
[d]Defined as having any of the following adverse birth outcomes: preterm birth, small-for-gestational-age birth, low birth weight, and perinatal mortality.
[e]Birth weight below the 10th percentile of the reference population for same gestational age at delivery and gender.
[f]Birth weight at or above the 90th percentile of the reference population for same gestational age at delivery and gender.
[g]Defined as Kotelchuck index of prenatal care score of one.
[h]The weekly rate of weight gain in the second and third trimesters was calculated as the total gestational weight gain minus the estimated weight gain in the first trimester (i.e., 4.4 pounds for underweight women, 2.2 pounds for normal-weight women, and 1.1 pounds for overweight/obese women) divided by the duration of pregnancy in the second and third trimesters (gestational age at delivery in weeks minus 13 weeks). Institute of Medicine recommended weight gain rates were used to classify women into the inadequate, adequate, and excessive categories.
[i]Defined as babies delivered as singleton births, head first, and at ≥ 37 weeks for nulliparous mothers.

number of women served in Lexington and Sumter counties during a nine-year period, which may have contributed to enrollment of high-risk women into the program and possible high levels of adverse outcomes. The null findings might indicate that the intensity of services provided to this high-risk population was low as a result of high recruitment levels.

There has been concern on the part of HS programs about not achieving program goals in terms of breastfeeding initiation.[12] We found that HS women were more than likely than non-HS women to have initiated breastfeeding in the hospital. Our findings on the positive effects of HS participation on WIC participation indicate the value of HS services, which may have a lasting impact on the health of mothers and infants. Because HS programs serve participants until 18 months after delivery, future studies should consider other innovative designs to examine the long-term effects of HS program participation on mothers and infants.

An important finding in our study was that HS women were more than likely than non-HS women to exceed the Institute of Medicine's recommendations for weight gain during pregnancy, suggesting the need for adding healthy lifestyle consultations to existing HS programming and incorporating healthy weight gain in pregnancy as a benchmark to assess program impact.

Overall, despite possible unmeasured confounding and misclassification, our findings have important implications for care providers and health policymakers in terms of how to narrow racial disparities in perinatal health by serving high-risk populations via community programs. AJPH

ABOUT THE AUTHORS

Jihong Liu, Longgang Zhao, Xingpei Zhao, Eric Mishio Bawa, Sabrina Karim, and Anwar T. Merchant are with the Department of Epidemiology & Biostatistics, Arnold School of Public Health, University of South Carolina, Columbia. Kimberly Alston is with Midlands Healthy Start, Prisma Health, Columbia, SC. Jun Tang is with the Division of Biostatistics, South Carolina Department of Health and Environmental Control, Columbia. Sara Wilcox is with the Department of Exercise Science and the Prevention Research Center, Arnold School of Public Health, University of South Carolina, Columbia.

CORRESPONDENCE

Correspondence should be sent to Jihong Liu, ScD, Department of Epidemiology & Biostatistics, Arnold School of Public Health, University of South Carolina, 915 Greene St, Columbia, SC 29208 (e-mail: jliu@mailbox.sc.edu). Reprints can be ordered at http://www.ajph.org by clicking the "Reprints" link.

PUBLICATION INFORMATION

Full Citation: Liu J, Zhao L, Zhao X, et al. Impact of a large Healthy Start program on perinatal outcomes, South Carolina, 2009–2019. *Am J Public Health*. 2023;113(5):509–513.

Acceptance Date: January 8, 2023.

DOI: https://doi.org/10.2105/AJPH.2023.307232

CONTRIBUTORS

J. Liu conceptualized the study, supervised the statistical analyses, wrote the first draft of the article, and critically revised the article. L. Zhao conducted the statistical analyses and contributed to the writing, interpretation, and revision of the article. X. Zhao prepared the data and contributed to interpretation and revision. E. Mishio Bawa conducted the literature review and contributed to the writing, interpretation, and revision of the article. K. Alston conceptualized the study, oversaw the data collection, contributed to interpretation and revision, and obtained the funding for the Healthy Start Program. S. Karim prepared the data, conducted initial data analyses, and contributed to interpretation and revision. A. T. Merchant advised on statistical analyses and contributed to interpretation and revision. J. Tang conducted data linkages and contributed to interpretation and revision. S. Wilcox contributed to the writing, interpretation, and revision of the article.

ACKNOWLEDGMENTS

This study was partially supported by a Prisma Health-Health Sciences Center transformative seed grant. The Midlands Healthy Start Program was sponsored by the Health Resources and Services Administration (grant H49-MC00072).

We acknowledge the assistance of Shy'Davia Baxley in the early stages of this project.

CONFLICTS OF INTEREST

The authors report no conflicts of interest.

HUMAN PARTICIPANT PROTECTION

This project was approved by the institutional review board of the University of South Carolina and was declared as meeting the non–human participant criteria set forth in the Code of Federal Regulations.

REFERENCES

1. National Healthy Start Association. Healthy Start Initiative. Available at: https://www.nationalhealthystart.org/healthy-start-initiative. Accessed July 31, 2022.
2. US Department of Health and Human Services. Early childhood home visiting models: reviewing evidence of effectiveness. Available at: https://homvee.acf.hhs.gov/sites/default/files/2022-02/opre-homvee_summary_brief_feb2022.pdf. Accessed July 31, 2022.
3. August EM, Salihu HM, de la Cruz CZ, Mbah AK, Alio AP, Berry EL. A quasi-experimental design to assess the effectiveness of the federal Healthy Start in reducing preterm birth among obese mothers. *J Prim Prev*. 2015;36(3):205–212. https://doi.org/10.1007/s10935-015-0389-0
4. Cooper BP, Scharff DP, Elliott M, Rotter B. The impact of SLHS program on perinatal indicators. *Matern Child Health J*. 2013;17(6):1158–1165. https://doi.org/10.1007/s10995-012-1101-0
5. Kothari CL, Zielinski R, James A, Charoth RM, Carmen Sweezy L. Improved birth weight for black infants: outcomes of a Healthy Start program. *Am J Public Health*. 2014;104(suppl 1):S96–S104. https://doi.org/10.2105/AJPH.2013.301359
6. Vladutiu CJ, Mobley SC, Ji X, et al. A methodological approach for evaluating the Enterprise Community Healthy Start Program in rural Georgia: an analysis using linked PRAMS, birth records and program data. *Matern Child Health J*. 2021;25(10):1516–1525. https://doi.org/10.1007/s10995-021-03205-4
7. Salihu HM, August EM, Mbah AK, Alio AP, Berry EL, Aliyu MH. Impact of a federal Healthy Start program on feto-infant morbidity associated with absent fathers: a quasi-experimental study. *Matern Child Health J*. 2014;18(9):2054–2060. https://doi.org/10.1007/s10995-014-1451-x
8. Meghea CI, Raffo JE, VanderMeulen P, Roman LA. Moving toward evidence-based federal Healthy Start program evaluations: accounting for bias in birth outcomes studies. *Am J Public Health*. 2014;104(suppl 1):S25–S27. https://doi.org/10.2105/AJPH.2013.301276
9. Austin PC. An introduction to propensity score methods for reducing the effects of confounding in observational studies. *Multivariate Behav Res*. 2011;46(3):399–424. https://doi.org/10.1080/00273171.2011.568786
10. Lu MC, Halfon N. Racial and ethnic disparities in birth outcomes: a life-course perspective. *Matern Child Health J*. 2003;7(1):13–30. https://doi.org/10.1023/A:1022537516969
11. Lu MC, Kotelchuck M, Culhane JF, Hobel CJ, Klerman LV, Thorp JM Jr. Preconception care between pregnancies: the content of internatal care. *Matern Child Health J*. 2006;10(suppl 5):107–122. https://doi.org/10.1007/s10995-006-0118-7
12. Healthy Start EPIC Center. Summary of findings from the 2017 National Healthy Start Program evaluation. Available at: https://healthystartepic.org/wp-content/uploads/2021/05/2017-HS-Eval-Summary_Posted-May-2021.pdf. Accessed September 25, 2022.

Population Monitoring of SARS-CoV-2 Infections via Random Sampling During the COVID-19 Pandemic

Paul Elliott, PhD, Helen Ward, PhD, and Steven Riley, DPhil

ABOUT THE AUTHORS

All authors are with the School of Public Health, Imperial College London, London, United Kingdom. Steven Riley is also with UK Data, Analytics and Surveillance, UK Health Security Agency, London, United Kingdom.

See also Morabia, p. 462, Dean et al., p. 517, Jernigan et al., p. 520, Bendavid, p. 523, Pastor-Barriuso et al., p. 525, Pérez-Gómez et al., p. 533, and Elliott et al., p. 545.

AJPH May 2023, Vol 113, No. 5

As the COVID-19 pandemic took hold in early 2020, most countries were poorly equipped to deal with it. Despite the entreaties of the World Health Organization to "test, test, test,"[1] few countries had the infrastructure, test equipment, laboratories, or resources to implement wide-scale testing. With the growing realization that severe acute respiratory syndrome coronavirus 2 (SARS-CoV-2) infection could be transmitted by those with mild symptoms and genuinely asymptomatic individuals,[2] it became clear that relying on testing only symptomatic people who went to health services (and were able to get a test) would fail to interrupt a substantial proportion of transmission and would give a biased view of the pandemic.[3] Accurate data on the extent of infection in the community and defining who was most at risk (and where) were essential to plan for demands on health services and to guide public health action in the absence, at that time, of vaccines and effective treatments.

Against this background, some countries invested early in community-wide testing of random members of the population to identify people with current infection. They used swabs and RT–PCR (reverse transcription–polymerase chain reaction) to determine current infection or past infection by testing for SARS-CoV-2 antibodies. The aims were to monitor trends in SARS-CoV-2 infection at a population level; gain new epidemiologic knowledge of who was at risk, when, and where; and (later, through viral sequencing of positive swabs) provide early warning of new variants appearing in the population. Antibody prevalence could also inform estimates of cumulative community infection rates, particularly important in early waves, when there was limited capacity for testing those with mild cases or their contacts.

The Seroepidemiological Survey of SARS-CoV-2 Virus Infection in Spain (Estudio Nacional de Sero-Epidemiología de la Infección por SARS-CoV-2 en España; ENE-COVID; see Pastor-Barriuso et al. [p. 525] in this issue of *AJPH*), conducted from April 27 to June 22, 2020, during lockdown, demonstrated regional heterogeneity in prevalence, which was higher in central regions of Spain. Even in areas with a high burden from the first wave of the pandemic, only around 10% of participants had antibodies,[4] indicating that large numbers of people were still vulnerable to infection.

A subsequent round of data collection was added in November 2020 during the second wave of infections. This high-quality study addressed many of the elements required to provide reliable data on symptom reporting and antibody prevalence at a community level. At the time, policymakers were largely in the dark about the proportion of the population that had been infected with SARS-CoV-2 during the first and second waves. Data on symptoms, comorbidities, and other risk factors and antibody levels were obtained from a stratified random cross-section of the noninstitutionalized population of Spain. The aim was to provide reliable estimates of prevalence by key demographics, including information at the province level.

The first wave of the study included 68 287 participants (69.1% of eligible people) who received a point-of-care test (lateral flow immunoassay [LFIA] device) for SARS-CoV-2 IgG (immunoglobulin G) antibodies, with a more accurate laboratory immunoassay also being done. The investigators used study weights to adjust for any bias introduced by the sample design (including oversampling in relatively less-populated areas) and variable response rates in different subsections of the population. Local primary health care teams obtained data nationally using a common protocol to ensure comparability across areas. Sampling was done by household, with allowance made in the statistical analysis for clustering at the household level. Importantly, the very high response rate ensured that the prevalence estimates provided an accurate representation of the (cumulative) community prevalence of infection. Moreover, the large size and reach of the study, both regionally and by age (from infants to the elderly), meant that relatively precise estimates of prevalence for different demographic groups could be fed back to policymakers.

Meanwhile, in the United Kingdom, two large-scale studies with complementary designs were initiated to measure the prevalence of virus and of antibodies in random samples of the population: the REal-time Assessment of Community Transmission (REACT) Study in England[5] and the Office for National Statistics (ONS) COVID-19 Infection Survey (CIS) across the United Kingdom.[6] REACT included REACT-1, which tested for the virus by RT–PCR from self-administered throat and nose swabs, and REACT-2, which tested for antibodies using a self-taken LFIA test. Both were designed to be representative of the population of England as a whole; had wide coverage by age, sex, ethnicity, and small geographic area and region; used sample weighting to produce population estimates of prevalence; and aimed to provide rapid, unbiased, and authoritative information to the government, the scientific community, and the public.

The REACT-1 study ran for approximately two to three weeks every month over 19 distinct rounds from May 1, 2020 to March 31, 2022, giving a detailed and dynamic picture of the pandemic in England as it unfolded (Figure 1).[7] Overall, more than 2.5 million people aged 5 years and older took part. The REACT-2 study included more than 900 000 adults over six rounds from June 2020 to May 2021. The ongoing ONS–CIS survey used a random household design and tested both for virus through RT–PCR and antibodies using a laboratory ELISA (enzyme-linked immunosorbent assay) test following a blood draw.[8]

These examples from Spain and the United Kingdom were some of the earliest (and largest) to use community-based samples, but similar initiatives were developed in other national, regional, and local areas. In mid-2020, Serotracker was established, collating data on antibody prevalence to an interactive dashboard that monitors and synthesizes data from studies across the world.[9]

What have we learned from these studies and what are the take home messages for monitoring future outbreaks of severe respiratory infections?

1. Antibody prevalence following the first wave of the pandemic in the United Kingdom[10] and Spain[4] was approximately 6% to 10%, so the capacity for large subsequent waves was high.
2. Patterns of infection in the community were substantially different from patterns of cases or hospitalizations, and these differences were important for policy (e.g., children were key to the pandemic at certain times).
3. There were marked social inequalities in risk of infection (and hence hospitalizations and mortality) during the first wave,[3,10] with important implications for planning pandemic response to minimize such inequalities in the future.
4. Relying on the results of routine testing of symptomatic people is biased both by the unavailability of tests (at

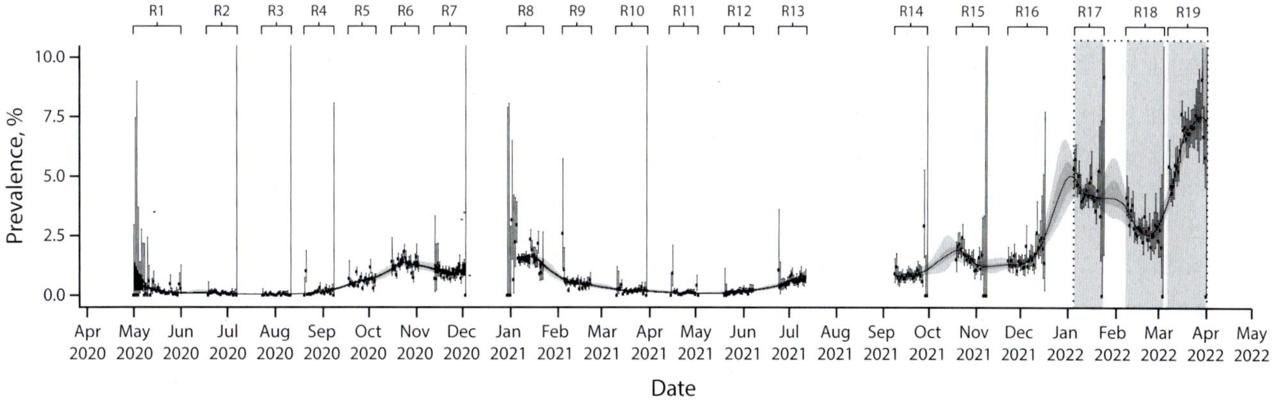

FIGURE 1— **Timeline and Weighted Prevalence of SARS-CoV-2 Infection: REACT-1 Study, England, May 1, 2020–March 31, 2022**

Note. REACT-1 = REal-time Assessment of Community Transmission-1. The figure shows the weighted prevalence of infection (black dots) and 95% credible intervals (vertical bars). P-spline model (black line) and 50% and 95% posterior credible intervals (dark and light gray shading) are fit to the data. Vertical gray-shaded areas represent "twin peaks" of Omicron BA.1 and Omicron BA.2 infections January–March 2022.
Source. Adapted from Elliott et al.[7]

least early in the pandemic) and by varying test-seeking behaviors in the community. Such data greatly underestimate the true infection rates because of the lack of comprehensive testing (in most countries) and the substantial numbers of asymptomatic infections.

5. ENE-COVID and REACT could make meaningful estimates of population case fatality rates, as they were able to include asymptomatic and mild infections in the calculations.[10,11]
6. Viral transmission did not occur equally everywhere but varied by place (and demographic groups) at different times,[3] with implications for public health measures to control infections.
7. Perhaps most importantly, most countries were massively ill prepared for the pandemic, and population testing and monitoring procedures (e.g., in the United Kingdom and Spain) had to be set up from scratch on an emergency footing.

The REACT and ENE-COVID studies showed that home-based self-sampling and testing is an efficient and effective way of carrying out mass testing at scale even during a lockdown. We now have a very clear picture of the requirements for situational awareness during a respiratory virus pandemic. Surely if we have learned one lesson, it is that we must invest, plan, and be much better prepared for future similar events. AJPH

CORRESPONDENCE

Correspondence should be sent to Professor Paul Elliott, School of Public Health, Imperial College London, St Mary's Campus, London W2 1PG, UK (e-mail: p.elliott@imperial.ac.uk). Reprints can be ordered at http://www.ajph.org by clicking the "Reprints" link.

PUBLICATION INFORMATION

Full Citation: Elliott P, Ward H, Riley S. Population monitoring of SARS-CoV-2 infections via random sampling during the COVID-19 pandemic. *Am J Public Health*. 2023;113(5):514–516.

Acceptance Date: January 7, 2023.

DOI: https://doi.org/10.2105/AJPH.2023.307231

CONTRIBUTORS

P. Elliott drafted the editorial. H. Ward and S. Riley provided edits and comments.

ACKNOWLEDGMENTS

The authors acknowledge funding from the Department of Health and Social Care in England for the REal-time Assessment of Community Transmission-1 (REACT-1) and REACT-2 studies.

CONFLICTS OF INTEREST

P. Elliott (director and principal investigator), S. Riley, and H. Ward (coinvestigators), with other team members, established the REACT-1 and REACT-2 studies of SARS-CoV-2 infection in the population of England. S. Riley is Director General of Data, Analytics and Surveillance at the UK Health Security Agency.

REFERENCES

1. World Health Organization. Laboratory testing strategy recommendations for COVID-19. March 21, 2020. Available at: https://apps.who.int/iris/bitstream/handle/10665/331509/WHO-COVID-19-lab_testing-2020.1-eng.pdf. Accessed December 16, 2022.
2. Mizumoto K, Kagaya K, Zarebski A, Chowell G. Estimating the asymptomatic proportion of coronavirus disease 2019 (COVID-19) cases on board the *Diamond Princess* cruise ship, Yokohama, Japan, 2020. *Euro Surveill.* 2020;25(10):2000180. [Erratum in: *Euro Surveill.* 2020;25(22)]. https://doi.org/10.2807/1560-7917.ES.2020.25.10.2000180
3. Riley S, Ainslie KEC, Eales O, et al. Resurgence of SARS-CoV-2 in England: detection by community antigen surveillance. *Science.* 2021;372(6545):990–995. https://doi.org/10.1126/science.abf0874
4. Pollán M, Pérez-Gómez B, Pastor-Barriuso R, et al. Prevalence of SARS-CoV-2 in Spain (ENE-COVID): a nationwide, population-based seroepidemiological study. *Lancet.* 2020;396(10250):535–544. https://doi.org/10.1016/S0140-6736(20)31483-5
5. Riley S, Atchison C, Ashby D, et al. REal-time Assessment of Community Transmission (REACT) of SARS-CoV-2 virus: study protocol. *Wellcome Open Res.* 2021;5:200. https://doi.org/10.12688/wellcomeopenres.16228.2
6. ISRCTN Registry. COVID-19 infection survey of the UK general population. ISRCTN21086382. Available at: https://www.isrctn.com/ISRCTN21086382. Accessed January 19, 2023. https://doi.org/10.1186/ISRCTN21086382
7. Elliott P, Eales O, Steyn N, et al. Twin peaks: the omicron SARS-CoV-2 BA.1 and BA.2 epidemics in England. *Science.* 2022;376(6600):eabq4411. https://doi.org/10.1126/science.abq4411
8. Office for National Statistics. Coronavirus (COVID-19) infection survey, UK statistical bulletins. Available at: https://www.ons.gov.uk/peoplepopulationandcommunity/healthandsocialcare/conditionsanddiseases/bulletins/coronaviruscovid19infectionsurveypilot/previousReleases. Accessed December 16, 2022.
9. Arora RK, Joseph A, Van Wyk J, et al. SeroTracker: a global SARS-CoV-2 seroprevalence dashboard. *Lancet Infect Dis.* 2021;21(4):e75–e76. https://doi.org/10.1016/S1473-3099(20)30631-9
10. Ward H, Atchison C, Whitaker M, et al. SARS-CoV-2 antibody prevalence in England following the first peak of the pandemic. *Nat Commun.* 2021;12(1):905. https://doi.org/10.1038/s41467-021-21237-w
11. Pastor-Barriuso R, Pérez-Gómez B, Hernán MA, et al. Infection fatality risk for SARS-CoV-2 in community dwelling population of Spain: nationwide seroepidemiological study. *BMJ.* 2020;371:m4509. https://doi.org/10.1136/bmj.m4509

Serological Studies and the Value of Information

Natalie E. Dean, PhD, David H. Howard, PhD, and Benjamin A. Lopman, PhD

ABOUT THE AUTHORS

Natalie E. Dean, David H. Howard, and Benjamin A. Lopman are with the Rollins School of Public Health, Emory University, Atlanta, GA.

See also Morabia, p. 462, Elliott et al., p. 514, Jernigan et al., p. 520, Bendavid, p. 523, Pastor-Barriuso et al., p. 525, Pérez-Gómez et al., p. 533, and Elliott et al., p. 545.

In this issue of AJPH, Pastor-Barriuso et al. (p. 525) describe the design and implementation of the ENE-COVID study—a nationally representative, population-based, longitudinal survey of severe acute respiratory syndrome coronavirus 2 (SARS-CoV-2) antibodies in Spain. Throughout the pandemic, serological surveys have been extraordinarily valuable for understanding COVID's epidemiology. In spring 2020—when ENE-COVID conducted its first survey phase—diagnostic tests were scarce, and there were important questions about the severity of SARS-CoV-2 and the extent of immunity after the first wave. Although conveniently sampled antibody studies from other countries provided rapid insights, these were not always reliable or adequately representative.[1] The ENE-COVID study stands out for its size (> 68 000 participants in the first phase), breadth (first serosurvey to capture the entire age range, from babies to adults older than 90 years), and rigor (stratified two-stage probability sampling design).

The ENE-COVID study provided value locally, nationally, and internationally. The study was designed to provide sufficiently precise estimates of cumulative incidence of infection for each province in the country. Region-specific estimates enabled policymakers to "delineat[e] different schedules for recovering activity across the country" (although it turned out that all areas had seroprevalence well below any herd immunity threshold). At the national level, the study captured age-specific seroprevalence and risk factors for infection.[2] Seroprevalence was similar in men and women, in contrast to national surveillance data depicting differing burden. Globally, the study generated results that were impactful as they contributed to broader epidemiological understanding of the new pathogen. The severity of SARS-CoV-2 was unknown early in the pandemic, making it difficult for policymakers to formulate a response. ENE-COVID provided early, reliable insights on the proportion of infections that were asymptomatic.[2]

It is a useful exercise to reflect back on surveillance studies such as ENE-COVID and define the elements that added value. Which outputs of this and similar studies were most impactful for local, national, and international decision-making? What made these outputs especially valuable—rigor, representativeness, timeliness? And how did the value of these outputs evolve and the studies adapt throughout the course of the pandemic? Such a reflective exercise is important for planning future surveillance activities for SARS-CoV-2 and other pathogens.

The concept of the "value of information," which draws from the fields of economics[3] and decision science, is a useful framework here. One natural application in infectious disease epidemiology is infectious disease modeling. Surveillance data are piped into models as parameters or data streams for calibration, and these models are used for making projections or for scenario modeling (i.e., comparing the potential impact of different policies).[4] A logical question then is whether higher-resolution surveillance data translate to better projections or scenario comparisons. This question can be examined by running the model with different data inputs and looking for qualitative changes in the conclusions. Even more challenging to address, though, is whether policymakers demand a certain level of precision for decision-making. During the pandemic, modelers working within public health agencies described incredibly rapid turnaround times, too short for computationally complex models. Nimble models can be better-suited in these settings.

Importantly, the value of surveillance data is not constant over time and space. Data generation, like other investments, can occasionally have diminishing returns. At the beginning of the COVID-19 pandemic, studies were needed to establish basic epidemiological quantities. Field work for ENE-COVID started less than four weeks after the survey was identified as a national priority in Spain, and the first wave of data collection was completed in two weeks.[5] In contrast to data that are globally valuable, local data can be impactful because of the anecdotal weight it carries (here are actual infections that have occurred within the community), but it can also be redundant. Does the same study need to be replicated across all regions? For ENE-COVID, were province-specific estimates of seroprevalence needed, or was the key estimand the *underreporting ratio*, which could be measured in fewer locations but then used to extrapolate local burden from case reports? Would extrapolated estimates have been "good enough" for decision-making? And would cutting down on the complexity in one dimension (i.e., number of provinces) have enabled the study to expand in another dimension (i.e., number of rounds of sampling, adding in polymerase chain reaction [PCR] swabbing for active infection)?

Tracking cumulative incidence over time is useful, but even better is to consider: "What data should we collect next to narrow down the decision space?" The experiences of the COVID-19 pandemic emphasize the importance of flexibility and adaptability in studies. The key questions evolved over time,[6] from establishing basic epidemiological characteristics to assessing the effectiveness of different policies, or measuring the durability of antibodies in previously infected individuals. The end of one study serves as a starting point for the next—it is a pool of seronegative participants for an incidence cohort, or a pool of seropositive participants for an antibody waning cohort. Although the ENE-COVID study did not extend into the period when vaccines were widely deployed, large studies like the United Kingdom's Office for National Statistics (ONS) COVID-19 Infection Survey have addressed "vaccine-era" questions. They characterized population levels of immunity conferred by previous infection, immunity via vaccination, and "hybrid immunity" in vaccinated and infected individuals (quantities that are difficult to disentangle without serosurveys). When the omicron variant emerged, there was a need to revisit basic epidemiological questions (such as severity profile), but reinfections made antibody surveys difficult to interpret.[7] PCR swabbing for active infection made the ONS COVID-19 Infection Survey a critical resource to study the omicron variant—and the ONS is piloting adding influenza and respiratory syncytial virus testing to COVID-19 testing.[8] This sort of adaptation enables the study to maintain value while leveraging the extraordinary effort put into its initial design.

In the United States, we look to Spain and the United Kingdom in envy for their capacity to conduct such large, population-based studies. No such serosurveys of that size or representativeness were conducted in the United States, which we attribute to lack of integrated, national public health machinery with a strong community presence. Such levels of participation feel beyond reach here. Repeated cross-sectional studies of antibodies in US blood donors were helpful in characterizing changes in seroprevalence over time and by region,[9] but were constrained by their design—excluding children, for example. The studies could also not adapt to keep pace with evolving questions. One wonders what we lost by not having the same high-quality, locally generated insights.

Not all pathogens will be like SARS-CoV-2, but in a sense, the pandemic is the ultimate case study. We can put ourselves back in time, starting in spring 2020, acknowledging the enormous uncertainty about what the future would hold. Now, as the acute phase of the pandemic winds down, it's time to ask questions about what studies ought to be done in both "peacetime" and during a pandemic. How does better-quality information translate into better policy? A better-informed and trusting public? Better interventions? And can we use this information to design better surveillance systems? A systematic assessment of the serosurveillance studies that ran during the pandemic may be as good a place as any to unpack these questions. Our view is that ambitious and wide-ranging projects like ENE-COVID were the right studies for the moment at the beginning of the pandemic. But as the pandemic progressed, studies that evolved, such as those conducted by the ONS in the United Kingdom, were the most impactful. As epidemiologists, we must acknowledge that these discussions require policymakers, economists, modelers, and information theorists. The answers to these questions are large, unwieldy, and sometimes humbling, but the act of asking the questions can set us on the right track. As with the 1918 pandemic, we will be working to learn from the COVID-19 pandemic for a long time. AJPH

CORRESPONDENCE

Correspondence should be sent to Natalie E. Dean, 1518 Clifton Rd NE, Mailstop 1518-002-3AA, Atlanta, GA 30322 (e-mail: nataliedean@emory.edu). Reprints can be ordered at http://www.ajph.org by clicking the "Reprints" link.

PUBLICATION INFORMATION

Full Citation: Dean NE, Howard DH, Lopman BA. Serological studies and the value of information. *Am J Public Health*. 2023;113(5):517–519.

Acceptance Date: January 22, 2023.

DOI: https://doi.org/10.2105/AJPH.2023.307245

CONTRIBUTORS

N. E. Dean wrote the first draft, and all authors edited the editorial.

CONFLICTS OF INTEREST

The authors have no conflicts of interest to declare.

REFERENCES

1. Gelman A. Concerns with that Stanford study of coronavirus prevalence. Statistical Modeling, Causal Inference, and Social Science. 2020. Available as: https://statmodeling.stat.columbia.edu/2020/04/19/fatal-flaws-in-stanford-study-of-coronavirus-prevalence. Accessed January 19, 2023.
2. Pollán M, Pérez-Gómez B, Pastor-Barriuso R, et al. Prevalence of SARS-CoV-2 in Spain (ENE-COVID): a nationwide, population-based seroepidemiological study. *Lancet.* 2020;396(10250):535–544. https://doi.org/10.1016/S0140-6736(20)31483-5
3. Hughes-Cromwick E, Coronado J. The value of US government data to US business decisions. *J Econ Perspect.* 2019;33(1):131–146.
4. Cramer EY, Ray EL, Lopez VK, et al. Evaluation of individual and ensemble probabilistic forecasts of COVID-19 mortality in the United States. *Proc Natl Acad Sci U S A.* 2022;119(15):e2113561119. https://doi.org/10.1073/pnas.2113561119
5. Hernán MA, Yotti R. Two pandemics, two surveys in the United States and in Spain. *Am J Public Health.* 2021;111(3):414–415. https://doi.org/10.2105/AJPH.2020.306105
6. Koelle K, Martin MA, Antia R, Lopman B, Dean NE. The changing epidemiology of SARS-CoV-2. *Science.* 2022;375(6585):1116–1121. https://doi.org/10.1126/science.abm4915
7. Dean N. Tracking COVID-19 infections: time for change. *Nature.* 2022;602(7896):185. https://doi.org/10.1038/d41586-022-00336-8
8. Office for National Statistics. Influenza and other respiratory viruses pilot study: Coronavirus (COVID-19) infection survey summary. December 15, 2022. Available at: https://www.gov.uk/government/statistics/influenza-and-other-respiratory-viruses-pilot-study-coronavirus-covid-19-infection-survey-summary. Accessed January 19, 2023.
9. Jones JM, Stone M, Sulaeman H, et al. Estimated US infection- and vaccine-induced SARS-CoV-2 seroprevalence based on blood donations, July 2020–May 2021. *JAMA.* 2021;326(14):1400–1409. https://jamanetwork.com/journals/jama/fullarticle/10.1001/jama.2021.15161?utm_campaign=articlePDF%26utm_medium=articlePDFlink%26utm_source=articlePDF%26utm_content=jama.2021.15161

Learning From COVID-19 to Improve Surveillance for Emerging Threats

Daniel B. Jernigan, MD, MPH, Dylan George, PhD, and Marc Lipsitch, DPhil

ABOUT THE AUTHORS

Daniel B. Jernigan is the director for the National Center for Emerging and Zoonotic Infectious Diseases, US Centers for Disease Control and Prevention (CDC), Atlanta, GA, and is former deputy director for public health science and surveillance, CDC. Dylan George is the director of operations for the Center for Forecasting and Outbreak Analytics (CFA), CDC. Marc Lipsitch is the director of science for the CFA, CDC, and is director for the Center for Communicable Disease Dynamics, Department of Epidemiology, Harvard T. H. Chan School of Public Health, Boston, MA.

See also Morabia, p. 462, Elliott et al., p. 514, Dean et al., p. 517, Bendavid, p. 523, Pastor-Barriuso et al., p. 525, Pérez-Gómez et al., p. 533, and Elliott et al., p. 545.

AJPH May 2023, Vol 113, No. 5

As the SARS-CoV-2 virus (the causative agent of COVID-19) began rapidly spreading around the globe in the spring of 2020, existing surveillance systems were not robust or comprehensive enough to meet the tremendous need for real-time, representative characterization of both pathogen and disease. Confronted with these challenges in England, as described by Elliott et al. in this issue of *AJPH* (p. 545), an alternative, novel, and broadly applicable surveillance platform was established—the Real-time Assessment of Community Transmission-1 (REACT-1) study. This system was designed and purpose-built through a collaboration of public health officials, health care providers, academic modelers, mathematicians, statisticians, logisticians, and epidemiologists. The methods and execution of REACT-1 proved successful in maintaining situational awareness as reported in more than 15 publications and numerous public health reports, leading to meaningful policies and mitigations with significant positive public health impact.

Several design and methodological factors contributed to REACT-1's success and serve as examples for improving surveillance going forward.

- Bring It Home—During the nationwide lockdown in England, when clinics were closing and health care services were limited, REACT-1 brought the study to the people, where they lived, rather than attempting to implement at the point of testing and care. This helped to prevent collection bias introduced through opportunistic sampling among available patients at available clinics.
- Self-Serve—The study used a novel specimen accessioning approach by sending swabbing kits to volunteering individuals and families for self-collection, thus giving health care providers time to focus on patients in greatest need. Notably, this effort provided a more representative view of COVID-19, demonstrating the spectrum of infection among both symptomatic and asymptomatic persons and estimating the prevalence of infection with fewer biases from varying inclination or ability to be tested.
- Go Long—REACT-1 established repeated collections of specimens and data, occurring in 19 rounds of study, approximately every two to three weeks for almost two years. This sustained effort not only provided point-prevalence and cumulative incidence of infection, but also revealed broad trends of transmission and the emergence and growth rates of new variants over time and across the region.
- Go Large—The study was adequately powered for regular estimates of disease impact and virus evolution prevalence estimates at regional and subregional levels in England. To date, over 2.5 million swabs have been collected from over 14 million people invited to participate. The size of the sample allowed for a frequency of collection that was sufficient and timely enough to inform public health leaders to make evidence-driven decisions on mitigation measures.
- Level Playing Field—One important component of REACT-1 was the use of random sampling. The effort benefited significantly from access to patient records in the country's National Health Service (NHS), utilizing random cross-sectional sampling down to the local level. REACT-1 achieved a response rate of around 18% and utilized linkages to the NHS data. The representativeness of the study's sample uncovered important epidemiological trends in disease by age, race/ethnicity, socioeconomic status, and other health equity measures. These data

supported identification of disparities in infection risk as a major driver of racial/ethnic disparities in COVID-19 mortality. The design, frequency, and data completeness in the sample provided reliable inputs for modeling and forecasts of COVID-19 in the United Kingdom, in contrast to the use of case counts in other countries, whose interpretation was far more variable in space and time.[1]

- Versatile Player—Given the breadth and duration of the REACT-1 investment, its utility exceeded the primary intent for situational awareness and allowed for measuring multiple other public health outcomes. The platform provided vaccine effectiveness estimates specific for vaccine formulation, number of doses, and by predominant variant. Through additional consent and long-term record linkage, the platform also provided a profile of COVID-19 symptoms over time and was able to show evidence of reinfection and the degree of protection from natural infection and vaccination.
- Keeping Score—The results of each round of REACT-1 revealed the transparency of the program's processes and findings. The data were released quickly, publicly, and on a known cadence, and were reported in the media and used by senior decision-makers to guide COVID response policies. Routine and open data release streamlined clearance processes, managed expectations on updates to near real-time situational awareness, and maximized the benefit of the information to decision-makers and the public.

The costs and complex coordination of a platform like REACT-1 were appropriate and proportionate to the significant impact of COVID-19; however, it may be challenging to maintain the effort when no emergency is present, and it may be difficult to emulate in resource-limited settings, even during emergencies. The REACT-1 team improved logistics and, notably, lowered costs as the study progressed. Exploring options to optimize processes and further minimize costs for similar capabilities will be important if the lessons learned from REACT-1 are to be replicated in other locations.

The emergence and circulation of the SARS-CoV-2 virus revealed the foundational need for robust virological surveillance to detect, characterize, and monitor virus variants. Systems such as the SARS-CoV-2 Sequencing for Public Health Emergency Response, Epidemiology and Surveillance (SPHERES) in the United States and expansion of other global genomic sequencing networks were critical for informing public health interventions.[2,3] Going forward, a platform like REACT-1 could provide rich information on virus evolution and impact; at a minimum, however, specimen collection with virus genomic characterization at capable sentinel laboratories in strategic locations globally are needed to provide the first defense.

Other alternative approaches have been applied during the COVID-19 response for improving public health surveillance using byproducts of the data revolution and recent digital health trends.[4] These capabilities may allow resource-limited jurisdictions to jump over traditional methods to use newer data-only approaches for public health surveillance, such as event-based surveillance, social media monitoring, smartphone-based crowdsourcing, exposure notification, use of the Internet of Things, and wearable technology. Nonetheless, without a grounding of these efforts to the clinical and laboratory monitoring of emerging pathogens, they may be limited as nonspecific signals and trends.

Recently, the World Health Organization developed a Health Emergency Preparedness, Response, and Resilience (HEPR) framework, which seeks to improve detection and public health monitoring through "collaborative surveillance."[5] This initiative focuses on public health intelligence, surveillance of threats, improved laboratory capacity for pathogen and genomic surveillance, and better forecasting. Rather than a single, purpose-built system like REACT-1, collaborative surveillance calls for better linkage and coordination between existing epidemiological and laboratory systems in human and animal health to achieve a "mosaic" of community surveillance. Additionally, initiatives for data modernization are being implemented to address gaps that challenged the early COVID-19 response and improve data system readiness and coordination.[6]

The REACT-1 platform was a major accomplishment in collecting, analyzing, and informing essential information in a time of crisis. It provides major lessons learned on how to improve surveillance systems generally and especially during a pandemic. A clear question will be, how do we apply this approach and the lessons learned from REACT-1 into legacy surveillance systems during nonemergency situations? And how can we quickly ramp up similar efforts when needed again? The challenge will be to find ways of optimizing similar approaches in other locations within available resources. Hopefully, collectively we can rise to this challenge. AJPH

CORRESPONDENCE

Correspondence should be sent to Daniel B. Jernigan, MD, MPH, Director, National Center for Emerging and Zoonotic Infectious Diseases, Centers for Disease Control and Prevention, 1600 Clifton Rd NE, MS H16-5, Atlanta, GA 30329 (e-mail: djernigan@cdc.gov). Reprints can be ordered at http://www.ajph.org by clicking the "Reprints" link.

PUBLICATION INFORMATION

Full Citation: Jernigan DB, George D, Lipsitch M. Learning from COVID-19 to improve surveillance for emerging threats. *Am J Public Health*. 2023; 113(5):520–522.

Acceptance Date: February 12, 2023.

DOI: https://doi.org/10.2105/AJPH.2023.307261

CONTRIBUTORS

All authors contributed equally to this article.

ACKNOWLEDGMENTS

We thank Taylor Mann, Jennifer Layden, MD, PhD, and other colleagues in the CDC's Office of the Deputy Director for Public Health Science and Surveillance and the CDC's Center for Forecasting and Outbreak Analytics for their support and encouragement of data modernization efforts.

Note. The findings and conclusions in this report are those of the authors and do not necessarily represent the official position of the CDC.

CONFLICTS OF INTEREST

The authors declare no potential or actual conflicts of interest from funding or affiliation-related activities.

REFERENCES

1. Dean N. Tracking COVID-19 infections: time for change. *Nature*. 2022;602(7896):185. https://doi.org/10.1038/d41586-022-00336-8
2. Centers for Disease Control and Prevention. SPHERES—a national open genomics consortium for the COVID-19 response. Available at: https://www.cdc.gov/coronavirus/2019-ncov/variants/spheres.html. Accessed February 2, 2023.
3. Marcenac P, McCarron M, Davis B, et al. Leveraging international influenza surveillance systems and programs during the COVID-19 pandemic. *Emerg Infect Dis*. 2022;28(13):S26–S33. https://doi.org/10.3201/eid2813.212248
4. Whitelaw S, Mamas MA, Topol EJ, Van Spall HG. Applications of digital technology in COVID-19 pandemic planning and response. *Lancet Digit Health*. 2020;2(8):e435–e440. https://doi.org/10.1016/S2589-7500(20)30142-4
5. World Health Organization. Strengthening the global architecture for health emergency preparedness, response and resilience. Available at: https://www.who.int/publications/m/item/strengthening-the-global-architecture-for-health-emergency-preparedness-response-and-resilience. Accessed February 2, 2021.
6. Centers for Disease Control and Prevention. Data Modernization Initiative. Available at: https//www.cdc.gov/surveillance/data-modernization/index.html. Accessed February 2, 2023.

Seroprevalence Studies Are Critical Early Pandemic Tools, and They Were Underappreciated During COVID-19

Eran Bendavid, MD, MS

ABOUT THE AUTHOR

Eran Bendavid is with the School of Medicine, Stanford University, Stanford CA.

See also Morabia, p. 462, Elliott et al., p. 514, Dean et al., p. 517, Jernigan et al., p. 520, Pastor-Barriuso et al., p. 525, Pérez-Gómez et al., p. 533, and Elliott et al., p. 545.

The early days of the COVID-19 pandemic were a period of great concern and urgent action. In short order, the virus that spread in Wuhan, China overwhelmed Bergamo, Italy's hospital system and was quickly making its way across borders and continents. The mobilization of the scientific and public health communities was commensurate with the challenge. Within weeks of the initial reports, the genetic structure of the virus was sequenced, opening the door for diagnostics and vaccine developments. Within a year, at least four vaccines were deployed, and more than 200 000 scientific articles focused on COVID-19 were published.[1]

In the remarkable explosion of scientific productivity, seroprevalence studies stand out as notably underrepresented. Not that seroprevalence studies were not done. Some were done and reported. However, the information obtained from seroprevalence studies was so critical for understanding the evolution of the pandemic that the existing studies seem notably sparse.

Why were seroprevalence studies so critical? The headline reasons are familiar: the reported number of cases were grossly undercounting the total number of infections; because the cases represented the ailing and those seeking medical care, the visible pandemic was not a trustworthy representation of the true pandemic absent seroprevalence studies. Molecular diagnostics were hard to come by in the early days of the pandemic, and testing in hospitals made the virus appear to be particularly lethal. Seroprevalence testing was needed to understand the true extent of infection spread in the population. At a basic level, this was a central piece of information for two fundamental measures: feasibility of herd immunity, and the infection fatality rate. Herd immunity is that theoretical threshold at which there are enough circulating members of the population immune to the infection that further spread is effectively halted. The infection fatality rate is the proportion of those infected that die from the disease. Both of these measures require knowing the true extent of infection spread and cannot be estimated from case numbers.

There are other fundamental reasons for prioritizing seroprevalence studies, beyond the feasibility of herd immunity and the infection fatality rate. First, they enable fundamental understanding of infection dynamics in subgroups, such as in different ages or by sex. Imagine the importance for school reopening decisions of clear knowledge about transmission rates among primary school-age children. Or having a clear sense of the age gradient in infection fatality rate. Such 1000-fold differences in fatality rates between the young and old should have been a real call to action for prioritizing protective public health measures. Finally, repeated seroprevalence studies open a unique window on how transmission risk evolves in the population and point to key drivers of infection such as occupation.

Nothing can substitute for seroprevalence studies. And no other study provides such foundational information for understanding the epidemiology and informing policy. For those reasons, the 40 or 50 seroprevalence studies conducted in 20 to 30 countries early in the pandemic were woefully scarce.[2] Perhaps as many at 150 countries did not have regional studies, let alone national seroprevalence studies.

In this issue of *AJPH*, Pastor-Barriuso et al. (p. 525) provide a summary of the ENE-COVID (Estudio Nacional de Sero-Epidemiología de la Infección por SARS-CoV-2) seroprevalence studies conducted in Spain between April and November 2020. With support from the Ministry of Health, the ENE-COVID provided ongoing and nationally representative information in near-real time early in the pandemic. The results of the early

ENE-COVID studies were published for the broader scientific community, and the findings, with nearly three years of hindsight, are published here.

The findings provide a unique lens on the evolution of COVID-19 in Spain during those early months of the pandemic. It is a fascinating story. We see how, in Spain, risk of infection shifted from those with high socioeconomic status in April to those with lower socioeconomic status by November. Prior to April, it was the well-heeled globe-trotting travelers that got infected. Following the lockdowns, it was the cleaners and caregivers that got infected and continued to fuel transmission. We also see where infections happened: inside the home. Living with an infected person was the greatest risk factor for testing positive.

In some ways, this is the oldest story in epidemiology. Those with greater means take greater measures to protect themselves, leaving those with fewer means who live in more crowded households to bear the risk of staffing grocery stores, delivering Amazon packages, continuing essential construction, and getting infected. This is how health disparities come into existence. The ENE-COVID studies shed a bright spotlight on this process.

Why were studies like ENE-COVID rare? If the information they provide is so central to understanding the epidemic and informing policy, why were they not prioritized by every government? The first national seroprevalence study conducted in the United States under the auspices of the Centers for Disease Control and Prevention was not done until September 2020.[3] Several reasons are readily available. Measuring seroprevalence at a national scale is costly. Even during nonpandemic times, a lot of coordination is required to test a nationally representative sample. The backroom operations behind the ENE-COVID study were undoubtedly massive. And some early seroprevalence studies generated backlash, which may have disincentivized interested investigators.[4]

There is one more reason. If the story in the ENE-COVID study is universal, then the poor stood to gain the most from scientific studies that made it hard to ignore the fact that existing policies were likely shifting the burden from those with greater means to those with less. And the scientific establishment—by and large well-to-do and highly educated—did not prioritize that evidence. Modeling studies arguing for lockdown policies were highlighted and prioritized for policy setting.[5] Those are easier to handle—even when shown to be problematic.[6,7] It is harder to acknowledge that policies that protect scientists and the wealthy are also hurting the poor.

The importance of the ENE-COVID study cannot be understated as public health systems retool and develop plans for future outbreaks. The confluence of scientific and government support for the study is inspiring. No study is perfect, but ENE-COVID's sample—large and largely representative—techniques, and science-sharing ethic are a playbook recipe for future planning. We all have much to learn from their experience. AJPH

CORRESPONDENCE

Correspondence should be sent to Eran Bendavid (e-mail: ebd@stanford.edu). Reprints can be ordered at http://www.ajph.org by clicking the "Reprints" link.

PUBLICATION INFORMATION

Full Citation: Bendavid E. Seroprevalence studies are critical early pandemic tools, and they were underappreciated during COVID-19. *Am J Public Health*. 2023;113(5):523–524.

Acceptance Date: February 12, 2023.

DOI: https://doi.org/10.2105/AJPH.2023.307259

CONFLICTS OF INTEREST

The author has no conflicts of interest to declare.

REFERENCES

1. Ioannidis JPA, Salholz-Hillel M, Boyack KW, Baas J. The rapid, massive growth of COVID-19 authors in the scientific literature. Royal Society Open Science. Available at: https://royalsocietypublishing.org/doi/10.1098/rsos.210389. Accessed December 29, 2021.
2. Ioannidis JPA. Infection fatality rate of COVID-19 inferred from seroprevalence data. *Bull World Health Organ*. 2021;99(1):19F–33F. https://doi.org/10.2471/BLT.20.265892
3. Bajema KL, Wiegand RE, Cuffe K, et al. Estimated SARS-CoV-2 seroprevalence in the US as of September 2020. *JAMA Intern Med*. 2021;181(4):450–460. https://doi.org/10.1001/jamainternmed.2020.7976
4. Eisen MB, Tibshirani R. How to identify flawed research before it becomes dangerous. *New York Times*. July 20, 2020. Available at: https://www.nytimes.com/2020/07/20/opinion/coronavirus-preprints.html. Accessed February 5, 2023.
5. Flaxman S, Mishra S, Gandy A, et al. Estimating the effects of non-pharmaceutical interventions on COVID-19 in Europe. *Nature*. 2020;584(7820):257–261. https://doi.org/10.1038/s41586-020-2405-7
6. Soltesz K, Gustafsson F, Timpka T, et al. The effect of interventions on COVID-19. *Nature*. 2020; 588(7839):E26–E28. https://doi.org/10.1038/s41586-020-3025-y
7. Kuhbandner C, Homburg S. Commentary: estimating the effects of non-pharmaceutical interventions on COVID-19 in Europe. *Front Med (Lausanne)*. 2020;7:580361. https://doi.org/10.3389/fmed.2020.580361

Design and Implementation of a Nationwide Population-Based Longitudinal Survey of SARS-CoV-2 Infection in Spain: The ENE-COVID Study

Roberto Pastor-Barriuso, PhD, Beatriz Pérez-Gómez, MD, Jesús Oteo-Iglesias, PhD, Miguel A. Hernán, MD, Mayte Pérez-Olmeda, PhD, Nerea Fernández-de-Larrea, MD, Marta Molina, MD, Aurora Fernández-García, PhD, Mariano Martín, MEng, Israel Cruz, PhD, José L. Sanmartín, MEng, José León-Paniagua, PhD, Juan F. Muñoz-Montalvo, MEng, Faustino Blanco, MD, Raquel Yotti, MD, and Marina Pollán, MD, on behalf of the ENE-COVID Study Group

See also Morabia, p. 462, Elliott et al., p. 514, Dean et al., p. 517, Jernigan et al., p. 520, Bendavid, p. 523, Pérez-Gómez et al., p. 533, and Elliott et al., p. 545.

Data System. The Spanish National Seroepidemiological Survey of SARS-CoV-2 (or ENE-COVID; SARS-CoV-2 [severe acute respiratory syndrome coronavirus 2] is the causative agent of COVID-19) was funded by the Spanish Ministry of Health, the Instituto de Salud Carlos III, and the Spanish National Health System.

Data Collection/Processing. A stratified 2-stage probability sampling was used to select a representative cohort of the noninstitutionalized population of Spain. ENE-COVID collected longitudinal data from epidemiological questionnaires and 2 SARS-CoV-2 IgG antibody tests. From April 27 to June 22, 2020, 68 287 participants (77.0% of contacted persons) received a point-of-care test and 61 095 (68.9%) also underwent a laboratory immunoassay. A second follow-up phase was conducted between November 16 and 30, 2020.

Data Analysis/Dissemination. Analyses use weights to adjust for oversampling and nonresponse and account for design effects of stratification and clustering. ENE-COVID data for research purposes will be available upon request from the official study Web page.

Public Health Implications. ENE-COVID, a nationwide population-based study, allowed monitoring seroprevalence of antibodies against SARS-CoV-2 at the national and regional levels, providing accurate figures by gender, age (from babies to nonagenarians), and selected risk factors; characterizing symptomatic and asymptomatic infections; and estimating the infection fatality risk during the first pandemic wave. (*Am J Public Health*. 2023;113(5):525–532. https://doi.org/10.2105/AJPH.2022.307167)

AJPH May 2023, Vol 113, No. 5

The Spanish National Seroepidemiological Survey of SARS-CoV-2 (Estudio Nacional de Sero-Epidemiología de la Infección por SARS-CoV-2, or ENE-COVID; SARS-CoV-2 [severe acute respiratory syndrome coronavirus 2] is the causative agent of COVID-19) is a nationwide population-based cohort study to quantify seropositivity for SARS-CoV-2 in the noninstitutionalized population of Spain.

DATA SYSTEM

ENE-COVID was conducted by the Spanish Ministry of Health and the Instituto de Salud Carlos III (ISCIII), in collaboration with the health services of all the Spanish regions (Autonomous Communities).

Purpose

The main aims of this longitudinal seroprevalence study were (1) to quantify the extent of SARS-CoV-2 circulation throughout the country during the first epidemic wave, (2) to monitor its evolution over time, and (3) to evaluate which factors were associated with greater risk of being infected by this virus. Because of the different patterns of evolution of the pandemic among Spanish regions, ENE-COVID's design was intended to provide accurate and representative estimates of the prevalence of infection at the province level.

Public Health Significance

ENE-COVID was carried out during the first and very severe epidemic wave of COVID-19 in a Spain under lockdown, at a time when diagnostic tests were scarce and the surveillance system was not yet able to give reliable data on the burden of SARS-CoV-2 infection. ENE-COVID tried to answer the 2 main questions associated with a pandemic: how many people were infected, and how many of them died?[1] Its results showed that, despite the high impact of COVID-19, the prevalence figures of infection were low, very far from what would be needed to support control measures relying on herd immunity. Also, having information on the intensity of the pandemic in each region contributed to delineating different schedules for recovering activity across the country. In addition, ENE-COVID provided reliable estimates of 2 basic public health indicators needed to evaluate and control the COVID-19 pandemic; namely, the proportion of asymptomatic infections and age-specific infection fatality risks.

DATA COLLECTION AND PROCESSING

ENE-COVID collects data from a sample representative of the overall noninstitutionalized population in Spain, through personal interviews and using 2 immunoassays (as explained in this section). To gather information about the evolution of the epidemic, 3 consecutive data collection rounds were carried out during a first phase of the study (April 27–June 22); a second phase, consisting of a unique round, took place in November 2020. Primary care staff from each of the regional health services carried out fieldwork (recruitment, epidemiological questionnaires, and antibody testing) under a common protocol developed by the National Center for Epidemiology at ISCIII.

The training of all personnel was coordinated via a Web platform established at the National School of Public Health at ISCIII. The National Statistics Institute (INE) provided the name, age, and phone numbers of all residents registered in the selected households. Regional call centers and health care centers tried to contact each household by phone on different days and at different times.

The first person answering the call was informed about the general purpose of the study. If they agreed to participate, an initial phone questionnaire collected and updated the information on the current residents in the house and on the characteristics of the household. All people living in each household were invited either to go to their primary health care center or to allow a home visit, during which they provided written informed consent. At that visit, primary care staff collected epidemiological data through computer-assisted personal interviews; these included a history of symptoms compatible with COVID-19 (fever, chills, severe tiredness, sore throat, cough, shortness of breath, headache, anosmia or ageusia, and nausea, vomiting, or diarrhea), contact with confirmed or suspected cases, and other risk factors. Participants also had a point-of-care rapid test to detect antibodies against SARS-CoV-2 and, optionally, donated a blood sample to assess the presence of IgG antibodies in serum with a more precise technique.

The Ministry of Health designed a secure Web application specifically for this study to save both questionnaire and point-of-care test results. Blood samples were centrifuged to obtain the sera, labeled, stored refrigerated at the primary health care centers, and sent to the laboratory every 2 or 3 days. Serum samples were analyzed either at the National Center for Microbiology (CNM-ISCIII) or in 1 of 28 selected regional microbiology laboratories under CNM-ISCIII coordination.

The study used 2 immunoassays: (1) a point-of-care test applied to finger-prick blood to detect IgG antibodies against the receptor-binding domain of SARS-CoV-2 spike protein (Orient Gene Biotech COVID-19 IgG/IgM Rapid Test Cassette, Zhejiang, China; reference GCCOV-402a), with a sensitivity of 82% to 93% and a specificity of 99% to 100% in preliminary validation studies at CNM-ISCIII and elsewhere[2]; and (2) a chemiluminescent microparticle immunoassay (CMIA) requiring venipuncture to detect IgG antibodies against SARS-CoV-2 nucleoprotein (SARS-CoV-2 IgG for use with ARCHITECT, Abbott Laboratories, Abbott Park, IL; reference 06R8620), with a sensitivity of 91% and a specificity of 99% in a meta-analysis of 23 diagnostic accuracy studies.[3]

Ethical Procedures

To allow the design and recruitment of a nationwide representative sample, a specific collaboration agreement was established between the Ministry of Health, the Instituto de Salud Carlos III, and the INE that regulated the access and use of personal data from the Municipal Register of Inhabitants. The ISCIII Committee for Ethical Research approved the study. The Spanish Agency for Personal Data Protection was consulted. All study participants provided written informed consent, with specific forms for adults, teenagers, parents of participating children, and guardians of mentally disabled participants. These documents were available in the 4 official languages of Spain. In addition, witnesses assisted participants who were not able to read any of them.

Population and Geographic Coverage

Target population. The target population was the entire noninstitutionalized household population of Spain according to the Spanish Municipal Register of Inhabitants, updated in January 2020. Residents registered in municipal rolls but without a health card were also included (public health care coverage is universal in Spain, but immigrants without residence permit are not registered). The study, however, excluded nearly 1.0% of the Spanish population residing in institutional settings, mainly care homes for elderly and disabled persons, health institutions, prisons, and military and religious institutions.

Sampling design. We used a stratified 2-stage sampling to select baseline participants in the ENE-COVID survey. Given the heterogeneous circulation of SARS-CoV-2 by Spanish region, the first level of stratification comprised the 50 Spanish provinces (47 mainland and 3 insular provinces in the Balearic and Canary Islands) and the 2 autonomous cities of Ceuta and Melilla. In addition, because SARS-CoV-2 transmission may be affected by population density, the second level of stratification corresponded to the municipality size, grouped into municipalities with fewer than 5000, 5000 to 20 000, 20 000 to 100 000, and 100 000 or more inhabitants. There were 185 nonempty population strata formed by cross-classifying provinces and municipality size groups. Within each stratum, we selected census tracts as first-stage sampling units and households within census tracts as second-stage sampling units. All residents in the household were invited to participate in the study.

Sample size determination and allocation to strata. We determined a total sample size of 90 000 people to obtain reliable estimates of SARS-CoV-2 seroprevalence in all Spanish provinces, accounting for design effect and potential nonresponse. To achieve a minimum sample size by province while preserving to some extent the population distribution, we assigned half of the total sample uniformly to the 50 provinces and 2 autonomous cities, and the other half proportionally to their population sizes. The sample allocated to each province was distributed proportionally to its population in the 4 municipality size groups. As a result of this sample allocation, persons from less populated provinces were oversampled to increase the precision of seroprevalence estimates in these regions. Thus, we calculated design weights as the inverse of the sampling fractions within each province to restore the actual population proportions when computing multiprovince estimates, either at the national level or by Autonomous Communities (first-level administrative division integrating 1 or several provinces).

Within-stratum sampling. To facilitate fieldwork and reduce sample dispersion, we selected participants within each stratum in 2 sequential stages. First, 1500 census tracts were randomly selected with probability proportional to their size; their geographical distribution is displayed in Figure 1. Afterward, we sampled 24 households within each selected tract by simple random sampling without replacement. All persons residing in the household were invited to participate in the survey (average household size = 2.50 residents),[4] yielding the target sample of 90 000 persons. All persons in any given population stratum had the same probability of being selected. The design effects, which were induced by correlated clusters of seropositivity among residents in the same household and households from the same census tract, inflate the variance of SARS-CoV-2 seroprevalence estimates, which were considered in statistical analyses. Further details of the ENE-COVID survey design are described elsewhere.[5,6]

Unit of Data Collection and Sample Size

Analysis unit. The unit of data collection and analysis was the participant. In the ENE-COVID survey, participants who completed the epidemiological questionnaire and received the point-of-care test were included in the point-of-care sample, and those who also donated a blood sample and received the CMIA constituted the CMIA sample.

Sample size. Of 98 886 eligible persons residing in 35 885 selected households, 10 238 could not be contacted and

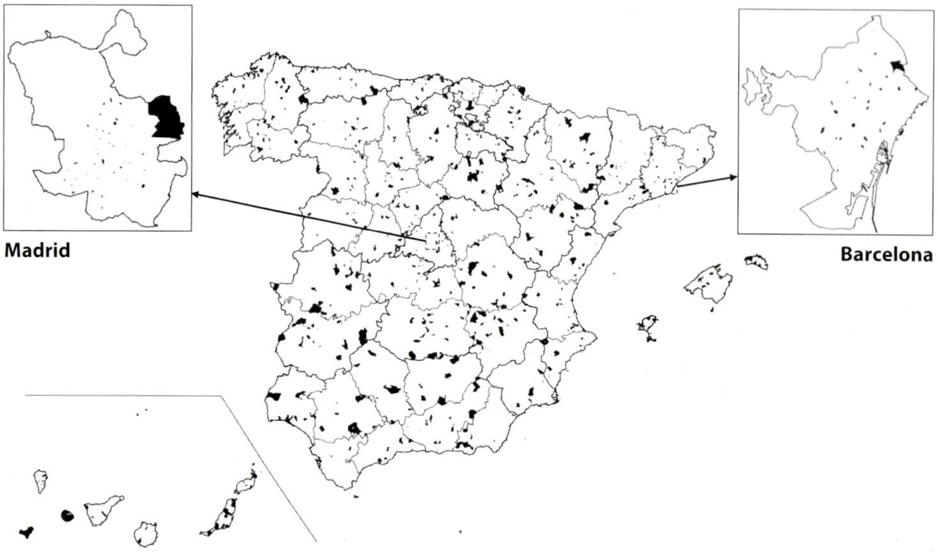

FIGURE 1— Distribution of Selected Census Tracts by Province in the Seroepidemiological Survey of SARS-CoV-2 Virus Infection in Spain (ENE-COVID): 2020

Note. Selected census tracts are represented by black areas. Census tracts selected in the largest municipalities (Madrid and Barcelona) are shown separately.

AJPH May 2023, Vol 113, No. 5

14 926 declined to participate (Figure 2). The point-of-care sample included 68 287 participants who received the point-of-care test in at least 1 of the 3 rounds during the first survey phase conducted between April 27 and June 22, 2020 (69.1% of eligible persons and 77.0% of contacted persons). Similarly, the CMIA sample comprised 61 095 participants who received this test in at least 1 round of the first survey phase (61.8% of eligible persons and 68.9% of contacted persons).

Response rates. Based on the sociodemographic characteristics of all eligible persons, response rates to the point-of-care test were lower among persons aged 25 to 29 years (59.3%) and older than 80 years (54.5%), among middle-aged men compared with middle-aged women (66.6% vs 73.3%), and among the lowest census tract income quartile (66.1%). Response rates for the CMIA evolved similarly to those for the point-of-care test by sociodemographic characteristics, except for a sharp decrease among those aged younger than 15 years (Figure 3). We used nonresponse weights to adjust for the different responses to the point-of-care test and the CMIA by gender, age group, and census tract relative income category.

Frequency of Data Collection

The first phase of ENE-COVID started 1 month after the peak of the first COVID-19 pandemic wave in Spain and included 3 successive follow-up rounds of data collection and serological testing between April 27 and June 22, 2020 (Figure 4). Each round was completed in 2 weeks, with a 1-week break between rounds. Half of the cohort was randomly assigned for data collection to the first week of each round and the other half to the second week, so that point-of-care testing and serum specimens were collected in all participants 2 to 4 weeks apart.

We conducted a second survey phase after the second wave of the COVID-19 pandemic, including a fourth round of data collection between November 16 and 30, 2020. All selected persons in the cohort were invited to receive the point-of-care test, whereas, in this round, the CMIA was only offered to a random subcohort of 200 census tracts as well as to participants with a positive result in previous rounds. More details are available in Spanish on the ENE-COVID Web site.[6]

Key Data Elements and Data Quality and Editing

The widespread geographical coverage, the large sample size of ENE-COVID, and the health situation of the country during the design, planning, and fieldwork implied relevant challenges about the feasibility, uniformity, and quality of the study. However, the study had

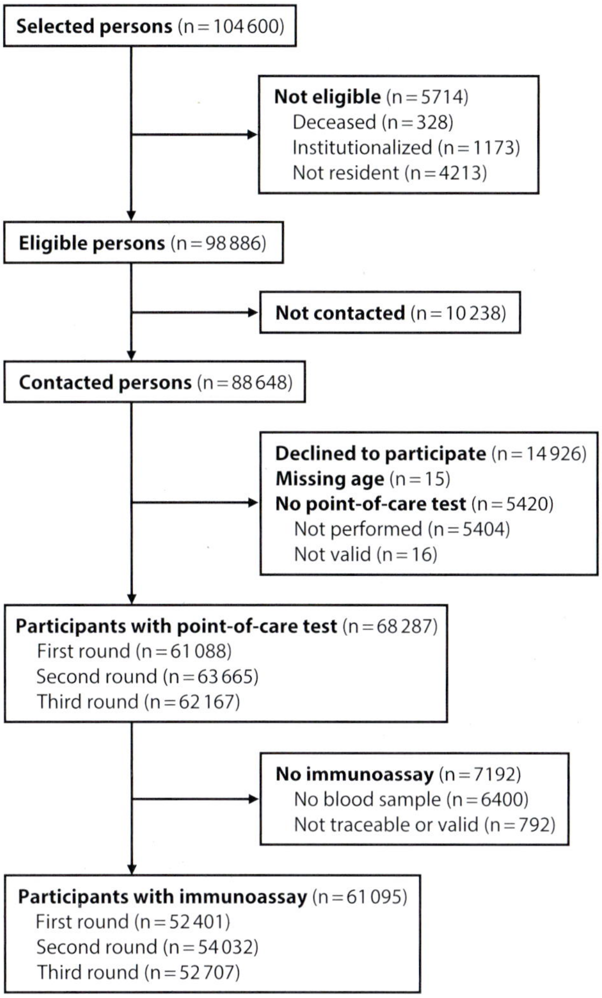

FIGURE 2— **Flowchart of Participants in the First Phase of the Seroepidemiological Survey of SARS-CoV-2 Virus Infection in Spain (ENE-COVID): April 27–June 22, 2020**

strong political support from health authorities, both at the national and regional level. Therefore, the leadership of the coordination team, the common protocol and Web-based training program, and the work of the very proactive and collaborative primary health care regional teams, in permanent contact with the central node to monitor fieldwork and information systems, favored the homogeneity and quality of the collected information. The epidemiological questionnaire included information on sociodemographic factors, COVID-19 symptoms, history of contacts, presence of chronic diseases, and other risk factors. Primary care staff collected this information before performing any serological exam, to avoid any influence of the test result on the participants' answers. Another key element is the good performance of the 2 tests used in ENE-COVID to measure SARS-CoV-2 IgG seroprevalence, selected by professionals from the CNM-ISCIII after performing specific validation assays of several candidate tests. Also, the use of a point-of-care test facilitated participation, allowing us to report the result to study participants immediately, whereas the CMIA allowed a more precise estimation, with a low risk of false positive results.

The continuous process of cleaning and curating the data registered during the computer-assisted personal interview started at the same time as the fieldwork. The electronic platform forced the study personnel to fill in all the questions included, thereby generating no missing data. The first phase of ENE-COVID included 3 contact occasions with the participants within a 2-month period (April 27–June 22), during which lockdown and restriction measures changed very rapidly. Therefore, the epidemiological questionnaire in each round added specific questions to explore risk of exposure, and again collected data on those variables that had quality problems. The information was checked, data between rounds were compared, and detected errors were corrected. Those participants that did not collaborate with ENE-COVID in any of the rounds have missing information for the round-specific data.

DATA ANALYSIS AND DISSEMINATION

In the sections that follow, we review elements of statistical analysis, interpretation issues, linkage ability, data release and accessibility, and provide key references.

Statistical Analysis

Sampling weights. Statistical analyses assigned sampling weights to survey participants to account for the different selection probabilities by province and the diverse response rates to the point-of-care test and the CMIA by

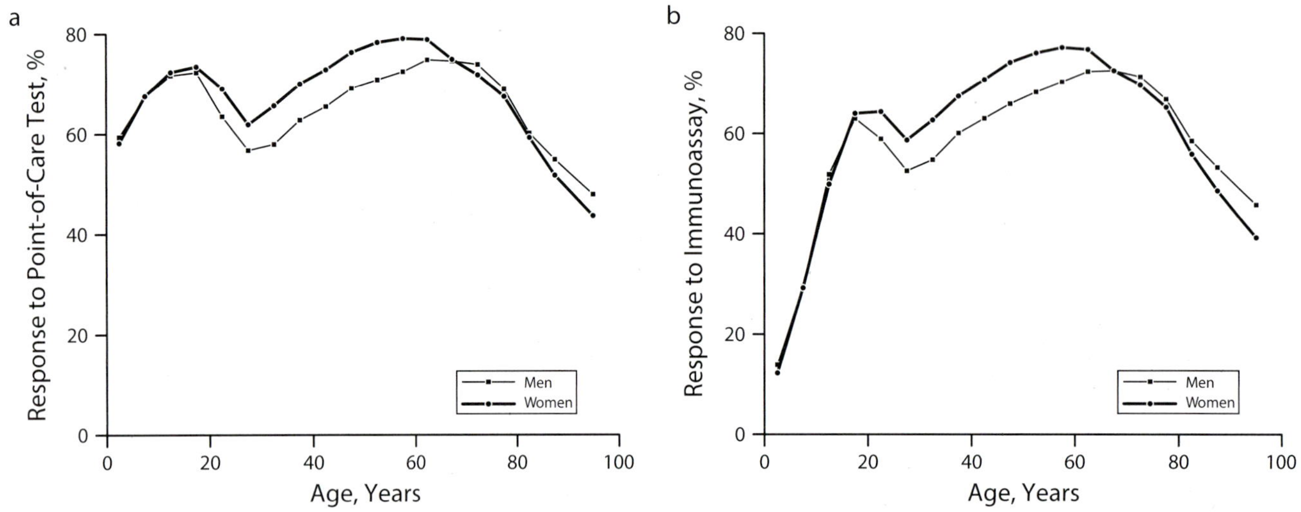

FIGURE 3— Response Rates to (a) Point-of-Care Test and (b) Chemiluminescent Microparticle Immunoassay by Gender and Age Group Among Eligible Persons in the First Phase of the Seroepidemiological Survey of SARS-CoV-2 Virus Infection in Spain (ENE-COVID): April 27–June 22, 2020

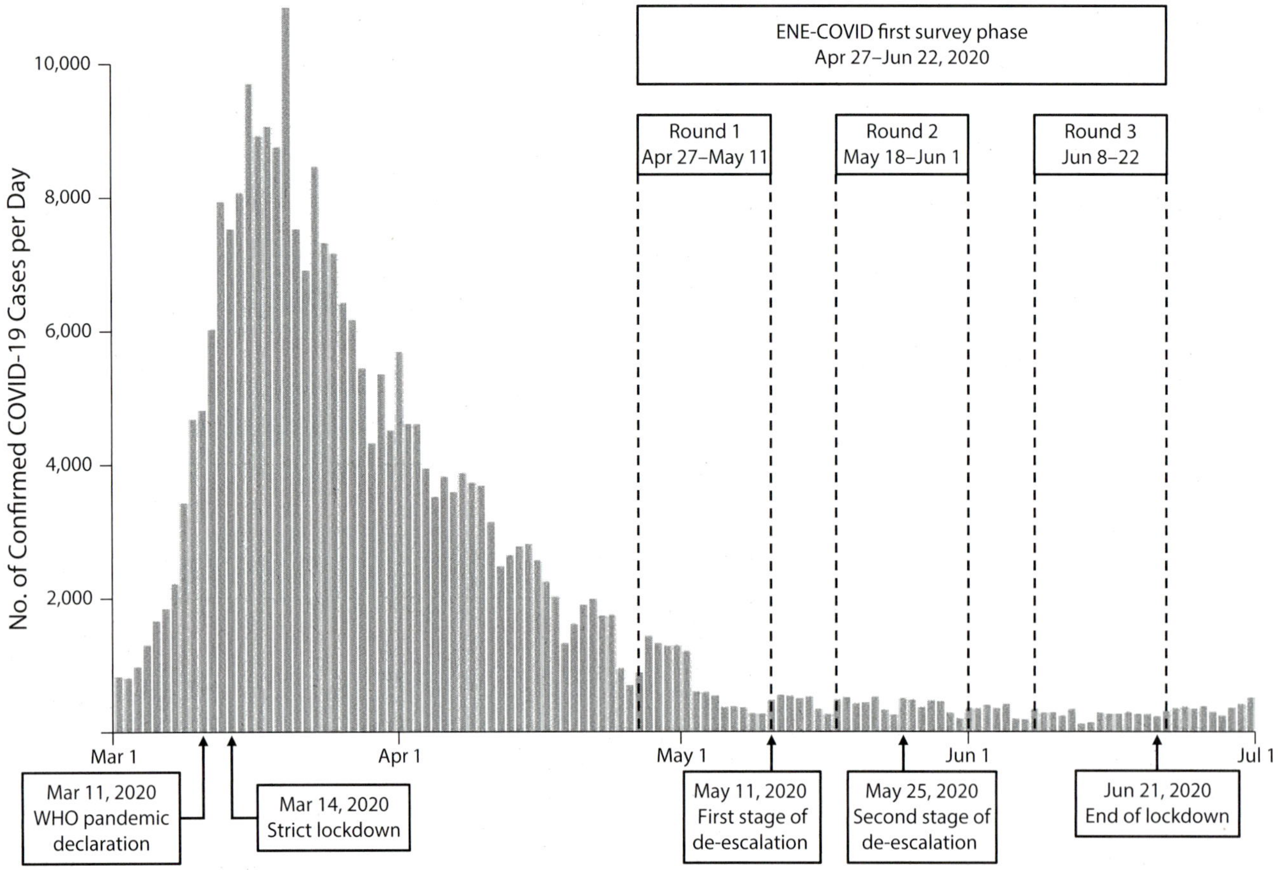

FIGURE 4— Follow-Up Rounds of Data Collection in the First Phase of the Seroepidemiological Survey of SARS-CoV-2 Virus Infection in Spain (ENE-COVID): April 27–June 22, 2020

Note. WHO = World Health Organization.

sociodemographic characteristics. Design weights were first calculated as the inverse of the selection probabilities within each province and municipality size stratum, which were then adjusted for nonresponse by poststratifying the sample by gender, 5 age groups, and 2 income categories, so that the weighted sum of participants in each stratum matched their population totals. Different sampling weights were calculated for the point-of-care and CMIA samples, and upper extreme weights (0.2% and 0.5%, respectively) were trimmed to prevent highly influential observations.

Design effects. Because of the complex survey design, the variance of SARS-CoV-2 seroprevalence estimates should consider stratification by province and municipality size and the clustering of seropositivity by household and census tract. The intratract correlation coefficient was 0.05 to 0.06, which inflated the variance of overall seroprevalence estimates by a factor of 3.93 for the point-of-care test and 3.90 for the CMIA. Finite population corrections could also be applied since the average sampling fractions of census tracts per stratum (6.6%) and households per census tract (4.9%) were not negligible.

Interpretation Issues

ENE-COVID had high participation rates, and the information available for nonparticipants allowed us to consider differences by age, gender, and census tract socioeconomic level to provide a reliable picture of the spread of the pandemic among the noninstitutionalized population in Spain. However, ENE-COVID left out institutionalized people, and the pandemic was particularly dramatic in certain nursing homes. No official register of this population was available at that time, and the study of these closed environments would have required a different approach.

As mentioned earlier under Frequency of Data Collection, a fourth round of ENE-COVID was conducted in the fall 2020 after the second pandemic wave with a slightly different design. The characteristics and results of this fourth round are described in our companion article in this issue of *AJPH* (p. 533) and can be consulted at the study Web page.[6]

Linkage Ability

ENE-COVID has individual data, whereas its design is based on households in selected census tracts, which have around 2000 to 3000 residents. This could allow researchers to perform spatial analyses based on their location, as well as to combine the data from this survey with contextual information from the Spanish census. In this sense, we have already profited from the ability to classify households according to the average personal income of the corresponding census tract. Also, the collaboration of the regional health services offers the future possibility of adding information from the clinical records of consenting participants.

Data Release and Accessibility

Very detailed national and regional reports, as well as interactive maps with the results for each phase of ENE-COVID, are available on the official study Web page, maintained by ISCIII (https://portalcne.isciii.es/enecovid19). This portal will also provide information on the official procedure of accessing ENE-COVID basic data for research purposes, which is being defined. Requests, which must include a short scientific protocol, will be assessed by the interinstitutional Collaborative Research Scientific Committee of ENE-COVID, as well as by the ISCIII Committee for Ethical Research, if necessary, to allow data use without compromising due confidentiality.

Key References

- Pollán et al.[5]
- Pollán et al.[8]
- Pastor-Barriuso et al.[3]
- Pérez-Gómez et al.[9]

PUBLIC HEALTH IMPLICATIONS

The first round of ENE-COVID served to characterize the geographical distribution of the first COVID-19 pandemic wave in Spain. It showed an important heterogeneity, with provinces with seroprevalences close to or greater than 10% mainly in the center of the country, contrasting with coastal regions and the islands, where prevalences were lower than 3%. Even in areas highly affected by the new pandemic, seroprevalence estimates were low, showing the difficulty of achieving herd immunity in the short term.

Contrary to what could be concluded from the information provided by the National Surveillance system,[7] seroprevalence was similar in men and women,[8] with no great differences observed by age group.[5,8] ENE-COVID was the first population-based study providing seroprevalence data from babies to people aged older than 90 years.

It was also the first population-based study estimating the proportion of asymptomatic infections,[5] and their distribution according to socio-demographic and epidemiological characteristics.[9]

The information provided by ENE-COVID and the number of deaths registered in our surveillance systems allowed us to estimate the infection fatality risk for SARS-CoV-2 in Spain.[3] The combination of serological and epidemiological information served also to monitor new infections during the 3 rounds of the first phase of the study, and propose a symptomatic risk score to predict COVID-19 among symptomatic people attended by primary health doctors.[9] AJPH

ABOUT THE AUTHORS

Roberto Pastor-Barriuso, Beatriz Pérez-Gómez, Nerea Fernández-de-Larrea, and Marina Pollán are with the National Centre for Epidemiology and the Consortium for Biomedical Research in Epidemiology and Public Health (CIBERESP), Instituto de Salud Carlos III (ISCIII), Madrid, Spain. Jesús Oteo-Iglesias, Mayte Pérez-Olmeda, and Aurora Fernández-García are with the National Centre for Microbiology and the Consortium for Biomedical Research in Infectious Diseases (CIBERINFEC), ISCIII. Miguel A. Hernán is with the Departments of Epidemiology and Biostatistics, Harvard T. H. Chan School of Public Health, Boston, MA. Marta Molina, Mariano Martín, José L. Sanmartín, Juan F. Muñoz-Montalvo, and Faustino Blanco are with the Deputy Directorate of Information Technologies, Ministry of Health, Madrid, Spain. Israel Cruz is with the National School of Public Health, ISCIII. José León-Paniagua and Raquel Yotti are with ISCIII.

CORRESPONDENCE

Correspondence should be sent to Marina Pollán, National Centre for Epidemiology, Instituto de Salud Carlos III, Monforte de Lemos 5, 28029 Madrid, Spain (e-mail: mpollan@isciii.es). Reprints can be ordered at http://www.ajph.org by clicking the "Reprints" link.

PUBLICATION INFORMATION

Full Citation: Pastor-Barriuso R, Pérez-Gómez B, Oteo-Iglesias J, et al. Design and implementation of a nationwide population-based longitudinal survey of SARS-COV-2 infection in Spain: the ENE-COVID study. *Am J Public Health*. 2023;113(5): 525–532.

Acceptance Date: October 29, 2022.

DOI: https://doi.org/10.2105/AJPH.2022.307167

CONTRIBUTORS

R. Pastor-Barriuso and B. Pérez-Gómez contributed equally to the article. R. Pastor-Barriuso, B. Pérez-Gómez, and M. Pollán were responsible for the conceptualization and design of the study. F. Blanco and R. Yotti were the executive coordinators of the project and led the relationship with regional health services. J. Oteo-Iglesias, M. Pérez-Olmeda, and A. Fernández-García were responsible for the validation of serological tests, coordination of microbiological laboratories, and acquisition of laboratory data. M. Martín, J. L. Sanmartín, J. León-Paniagua, and J. F. Muñoz-Montalvo were responsible for the study operation, including the coordination of data acquisition and logistics. M. Molina and I. Cruz developed the operational protocols for fieldwork and were responsible for training administrative and health personnel. R. Pastor-Barriuso, B. Pérez-Gómez, M. A. Hernán, N. Fernández-de-Larrea, and M. Pollán oversaw analyses and figures design. R. Pastor-Barriuso, B. Pérez-Gómez, and M. Pollán drafted the article and the remaining authors provided significant input, review, and editing. All authors read and approved the final version of the article.

ACKNOWLEDGMENTS

This work was supported by the Spanish Ministry of Health, the Institute of Health Carlos III (Ministry of Science and Innovation), and the National Health System, including the Health Services of all Autonomous Communities and autonomous cities: Servicio Andaluz de Salud, Servicio Aragonés de Salud, Servicio de Salud del Principado de Asturias, Servei de Salut Illes Balears, Servicio Canario de la Salud, Servicio Cántabro de Salud, Servicio de Salud de Castilla-La Mancha, Servicio de Salud de Castilla y León, Servei Català de Salut, Conselleria de Sanitat Universal i Salut Pública de la Generalitat Valenciana, Servicio Extremeño de Salud, Servizo Galego de Saúde, Servicio Riojano de Salud, Servicio Madrileño de Salud, Servicio Murciano de Salud, Servicio Navarro de Salud-Osasunbidea and Instituto de Salud Pública y Laboral de Navarra, Servicio Vasco de Salud-Osakidetza, and Instituto de Gestión Sanitaria. The Spanish Institute of Statistics provided the random selection of households and the information required to contact participants.

We thank all the nurses, general practitioners, administrative personnel, and other health care workers who collaborated in this study and all participants. This study is the result of the efforts of many professionals and the trust and generosity of more than 68 000 participants who have understood the importance of providing time, information, and samples to learn about the COVID-19 epidemic in Spain.

Collaborators of the ENE-COVID Study Group are listed in the Appendix, available as a supplement to the online version of this article at https://www.ajph.org.

CONFLICTS OF INTEREST

The authors declare they have no conflicts of interest.

HUMAN PARTICIPANT PROTECTION

The institutional review board of the Institute of Health Carlos III (ISCIII Committee for Ethical Research) approved the study (register no. PI 39_2020).

REFERENCES

1. Hernán MA, Yotti R. Two pandemics, two surveys in the United States and in Spain. *Am J Public Health*. 2021;111(3):414–415. https://doi.org/10.2105/AJPH.2020.306105
2. Hoffman T, Nissen K, Krambrich J, et al. Evaluation of a COVID-19 IgM and IgG rapid test; an efficient tool for assessment of past exposure to SARS-CoV-2. *Infect Ecol Epidemiol*. 2020;10(1):1754538. https://doi.org/10.1080/20008686.2020.1754538
3. Pastor-Barriuso R, Pérez-Gómez B, Hernán MA, et al. Infection fatality risk for SARS-CoV-2 in community dwelling population of Spain: nationwide seroepidemiological study. *BMJ*. 2020;371:m4509. https://doi.org/10.1136/bmj.m4509
4. Instituto Nacional de Estadística. Encuesta Continua de Hogares 2019. 2020. Available at: https://www.ine.es/prensa/ech_2019.pdf. Accessed August 24, 2022.
5. Pollán M, Pérez-Gómez B, Pastor-Barriuso R, et al. Prevalence of SARS-CoV-2 in Spain (ENE-COVID): a nationwide, population-based seroepidemiological study. *Lancet*. 2020;396(10250):535–544. https://doi.org/10.1016/S0140-6736(20)31483-5
6. Instituto de Salud Carlos III. National Study of SARS-CoV-2 Sero-Epidemiology in Spain (ENE-COVID). 2020. Available at: https://portalcne.isciii.es/enecovid19. Accessed August 25, 2022.
7. Centro Nacional de Epidemiología/Red Nacional de Vigilancia Epidemiológica. Análisis de los casos de COVID-19 notificados a la RENAVE hasta el 10 de mayo de 2020 en España. Institute of Health Carlos III. 2020. Available at: https://www.isciii.es/QueHacemos/Servicios/VigilanciaSaludPublicaRENAVE/EnfermedadesTransmisibles/Documents/INFORMES/Informes%20COVID-19/Informe%20n%c2%ba%2032.%20Situaci%c3%b3n%20de%20COVID-19%20en%20Espa%c3%b1a%20a%2021%20de%20mayo%20de%202020.pdf. Accessed August 25, 2022.
8. Pollán M, Pérez-Gómez B, Pastor-Barriuso R, et al. SARS-CoV-2 seroprevalence in Spain—authors' reply. *Lancet*. 2020;396(10261):1484–1485. https://doi.org/10.1016/S0140-6736(20)32266-2
9. Pérez-Gómez B, Pastor-Barriuso R, Pérez-Olmeda M, et al. ENE-COVID nationwide serosurvey served to characterize asymptomatic infections and to develop a symptom-based risk score to predict COVID-19. *J Clin Epidemiol*. 2021;139:240–254. https://doi.org/10.1016/j.jclinepi.2021.06.005

SARS-CoV-2 Infection During the First and Second Pandemic Waves in Spain: the ENE–COVID Study

Beatriz Pérez-Gómez, MD, Roberto Pastor-Barriuso, PhD, Nerea Fernández-de-Larrea, MD, Miguel A. Hernán, MD, Mayte Pérez-Olmeda, PhD, Jesús Oteo-Iglesias, PhD, Pablo Fernández-Navarro, PhD, Aurora Fernández-García, PhD, Mariano Martín, MEng, Israel Cruz, PhD, José L. Sanmartín, MEng, José León-Paniagua, PhD, Juan F. Muñoz-Montalvo, MEng, Faustino Blanco, MD, Raquel Yotti, MD, and Marina Pollán, MD, on behalf of the ENE–COVID Study Group

See also Morabia, p. 462, Elliott et al., p. 514, Dean et al., p. 517, Jernigan et al., p. 520, Bendavid, p. 523, Pastor-Barriuso et al., p. 525, and Elliott et al., p. 545.

Objectives. To describe participant characteristics associated with severe acute respiratory syndrome coronavirus 2 infection in Spain's first 2 COVID-19 waves per the Spanish National Seroepidemiological Survey of SARS-CoV-2 Infection (ENE–COVID).

Methods. A representative cohort of the noninstitutionalized Spanish population, selected through stratified 2-stage sampling, answered a questionnaire and received point-of-care testing April to June 2020 (first wave: n = 68 287); previously seronegative participants repeated the questionnaire and test November 2020 (second wave: n = 44 451). We estimated seropositivity by wave and participant characteristics, accounting for sampling weights, nonresponse, and design effects.

Results. We found that 6.0% (95% confidence interval [CI] = 5.7%, 6.4%) of Spain's population was infected by June and 3.8% (95% CI = 3.5%, 4.1%) more by November 2020. Both genders were equally affected. Seroprevalence decreased with age in adults 20 years and older in the second wave; socioeconomic differences increased. Health care workers were affected at 11.1% (95% CI = 9.0%, 13.6%) and 6.1% (95% CI = 4.4%, 8.5%) in the first and second waves, respectively. Living with an infected person increased infection risk to 22.1% (95% CI = 18.9%, 25.6%) in the first and 35.0% (95% CI = 30.8%, 39.4%) in the second wave.

Conclusions. ENE–COVID characterized the first 2 pandemic waves, when information from surveillance systems was incomplete. (*Am J Public Health*. 2023;113(5):533–544. https://doi.org/10.2105/AJPH.2023.307233)

AJPH May 2023, Vol 113, No. 5

When the World Health Organization declared the COVID-19 pandemic on March 11, 2020, Spain was among the most affected countries in Europe. On March 14, the Spanish government declared a state of emergency and a strict lockdown. Between April 28 and June 21, restrictions were progressively lifted, with different measures taken by each of the Spanish regions (known as autonomous communities).

Between January and April 2020, the National Epidemiological Surveillance System registered approximately 220 000 COVID-19 cases,[1] an underestimate because of limited availability of diagnostic tests, which were reserved for those with severe illness and symptomatic health care workers. To more accurately estimate the number of infected people, the Spanish COVID-19 Task Force proposed a nationwide, population-based seroepidemiological study in late March, and this was launched a few weeks later, in April 2020. A cohort of individuals was invited to participate in 4 rounds of the study. The first 3 rounds, with the first starting on April 27, took place during the first pandemic wave. The fourth round took place in November 2020, after the peak of the second pandemic wave at the end of October.

We used data from the nationwide seroepidemiological study to describe participant characteristics associated with severe acute respiratory syndrome coronavirus 2 (SARS-CoV-2) infection in the first 2 pandemic waves in Spain.

METHODS

The Spanish National Seroepidemiological Survey of SARS-CoV-2 Infection (Estudio Nacional de Sero-Epidemiología de la Infección por SARS-CoV-2 en España [ENE–COVID]) was a nationwide population-based cohort study to quantify the seropositivity for SARS-CoV-2 in the community-dwelling population of Spain.

Study Design and Population

We describe the study design in detail in our companion article (p. 525). Briefly, we selected 1500 census tracts and up to 24 households per tract through a 2-stage random sampling stratified by province and municipality size. We invited all residents in the 35 885 selected households to participate in the study. We collected serial data from epidemiological questionnaires and 2 serology tests (a point-of-care test and a laboratory immunoassay) from study participants in 2 survey phases. The first phase started 1 month after the peak incidence of the first COVID-19 pandemic wave in Spain and included 3 initial rounds of data collection at 3-week intervals between April 27 and June 22, 2020.

We conducted the second survey phase after the peak of the second pandemic wave and included a subsequent fourth round of data collection between November 16 and 30, 2020. Because of the comparable performance but easier implementation of the point-of-care test compared with the laboratory immunoassay during the first phase,[2] the laboratory test was offered in the second survey phase only to participants from a random subcohort of 200 census tracts stratified by autonomous community (first-level territorial division integrating 1 or several provinces; Figure A of the Appendix, available as a supplement to the online version of this article at http://www.ajph.org).[3]

To study SARS-CoV-2 seroprevalence during the first pandemic wave, we used the data of 68 287 participants who received the point-of-care test and 61 095 who received the laboratory immunoassay in at least 1 of the 3 rounds of the first survey phase (response rates were 69.1% and 61.8% among all eligible persons, respectively). To investigate new seropositive participants for SARS-CoV-2 during the second pandemic wave, we used the data of 44 451 participants who tested negative by all received point-of-care tests during the first phase and underwent such a test in the single round of the second survey phase (retention rate was 69.2% among all seronegative participants in the first phase by the point-of-care test). In addition, we analyzed new seropositivity by laboratory immunoassay during the second pandemic wave in 5045 participants of the random subcohort who tested negative by the laboratory immunoassay in the first phase and received that test in the second survey phase (retention rate was 92.1% among subcohort participants with negative immunoassays in the first phase).

Data Collection and Serology Tests

Trained staff from the Spanish regional health services collected data using a common protocol developed by the National Centre for Epidemiology of the Instituto de Salud Carlos III and the Spanish Ministry of Health. At each survey round, residents in selected households were contacted by telephone and invited to go to their primary health care centers or to allow a home visit. Residents who agreed to participate answered an epidemiological questionnaire on sociodemographic characteristics, risk factors, comorbidities, disability, symptoms compatible with having COVID-19, polymerase chain reaction (PCR) status, and contact with someone with confirmed or suspected COVID-19. Participants also received a rapid serology test and, optionally, donated blood samples for further laboratory analysis. The survey protocol is detailed in the companion article (in this issue of *AJPH*; p. 525) and is available in Spanish on the ENE–COVID Web site[3] and in a public repository (http://hdl.handle.net/20.500.12105/15247).

Briefly, the first serology test was a point-of-care rapid test applied to finger prick blood (COVID-19 IgG/IgM Rapid Test Cassette; Orient Gene Biotech, Zhejiang, China; reference GCCOV-402a) to detect the presence of immunoglobulin G (IgG) antibodies against SARS-CoV-2 spike protein; this showed a sensitivity of 82% and a specificity of 100% in a preliminary validation study.[2] The second test was a chemiluminescent microparticle immunoassay (CMIA) using serum samples (SARS-CoV-2 IgG for use with ARCHITECT; Abbott Laboratories, Chicago, IL; reference 06R8620) to quantify IgG antibodies against the SARS-CoV-2 nucleoprotein. Using a threshold of 1.40 for the sample to calibrator chemiluminescent signal ratio, the CMIA showed a sensitivity of 91% and a specificity of 99% in a meta-analysis of 23 diagnostic accuracy studies.[4]

AJPH May 2023, Vol 113, No. 5

Statistical Analysis

We estimated seropositivity for SARS-CoV-2 during the first pandemic wave as the proportion of participants who had detectable IgG antibodies against SARS-CoV-2 in any round of the first survey phase by the point-of-care test. We estimated new seropositivity during the second pandemic wave as the proportion of seronegative participants in the first phase who had detectable IgG antibodies against SARS-CoV-2 in the single round of the second survey phase by the point-of-care test. We calculated new seropositive participants by pandemic wave in a similar way for the laboratory CMIA based on a seropositivity threshold of 1.40; results are presented as sensitivity analyses because of the lower response rate to the CMIA and its limited application to a subcohort in the second survey phase. For each pandemic wave, we calculated seropositivity ratios (SPRs) by participant characteristics, taking the overall seropositivity of that pandemic wave as the reference.

We performed further analyses combining results from both tests to maximize either sensitivity or specificity. We estimated seropositivity for SARS-CoV-2 during the first pandemic wave as the proportion of participants who were found positive by either test (most sensitive approach) or by both tests (most specific approach) in the first survey phase. We estimated new seropositivity status during the second pandemic wave as the proportion of seronegative participants as determined by both tests in the first phase who were found positive by either or both tests in the second survey phase.

We assigned sampling weights to survey participants to account for the different selection probabilities by province and autonomous community and to adjust for the distinct response rates to the point-of-care test and the CMIA by gender, age group, and census tract income category. We used different sampling weights for the point-of-care test and the CMIA in each pandemic wave, and we trimmed upper extreme weights (0.2% to 0.5%) to prevent influential observations. All statistical analyses accounted for the effect of stratification and clustering of seropositivity by household and census tract on SE estimates. We calculated confidence intervals (CIs) using logit-transformed seropositivity estimates and log-transformed ratios and back-transformed CIs to the original scale for reporting, with design-based degrees of freedom equal to the number of first-stage sampling units minus the number of strata. We performed analyses using survey commands in Stata, version 16 (StataCorp LP, College Station, TX).

RESULTS

Figure 1 shows the geographical distribution of SARS-CoV-2 infection in the first and second pandemic waves. Table 1 presents seroprevalence figures together with seroprevalence ratios in each wave (Appendix Table A shows these figures separately in men

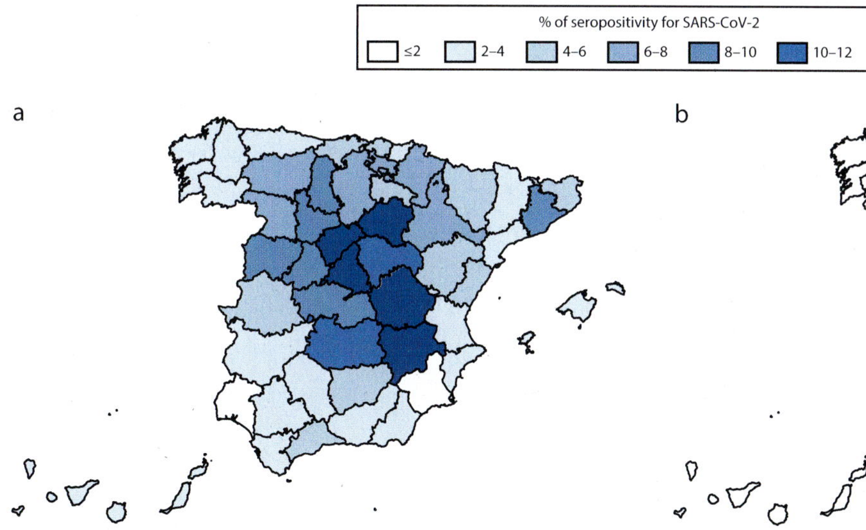

FIGURE 1— New Seropositive Participants for SARS-CoV-2 as Determined by the Point-of-Care Test in the (a) First and (b) Second Pandemic Waves by Province: ENE-COVID, Spain, April 27–June 22 and November 16–30, 2020

Note. ENE-COVID = Spanish National Seroepidemiological Survey of SARS-CoV-2 Infection/Estudio Nacional de Sero-Epidemiología de la Infección por SARS-CoV-2 en España; SARS-CoV-2 = severe acute respiratory syndrome coronavirus 2. The names of all Spanish provinces outlined on the maps are provided in Appendix Figure A (available as a supplement to the online version of this article at http://www.ajph.org).

TABLE 1— New Seropositive Participants for SARS-CoV-2 as Determined by the Point-of-Care Test in the First and Second Pandemic Waves by General Characteristics: ENE-COVID, Spain, April 27–June 22 and November 16–30, 2020

	First Pandemic Wave			Second Pandemic Wave		
Characteristic	No. of Participants[a]	Seropositivity,[b] % (95% CI)	Seropositivity Ratio[c] (95% CI)	No. of Participants[d]	Seropositivity,[e] % (95% CI)	Seropositivity Ratio[c] (95% CI)
Overall	68 287	6.0 (5.7, 6.4)		44 451	3.8 (3.5, 4.1)	
Gender						
Men	32 742	5.9 (5.5, 6.4)	0.98 (0.95, 1.02)	20 956	3.7 (3.3, 4.1)	0.98 (0.93, 1.04)
Women	35 545	6.1 (5.8, 6.6)	1.02 (0.98, 1.05)	23 495	3.8 (3.5, 4.3)	1.02 (0.97, 1.07)
Age, y						
0–19	12 581	4.0 (3.5, 4.5)	0.66 (0.59, 0.74)	7 543	4.0 (3.3, 4.8)	1.06 (0.92, 1.21)
20–34	9 552	5.1 (4.4, 5.8)	0.84 (0.75, 0.95)	5 217	4.3 (3.6, 5.1)	1.14 (0.98, 1.32)
35–49	16 051	6.4 (5.8, 7.0)	1.05 (0.98, 1.14)	10 427	3.6 (3.1, 4.2)	0.96 (0.85, 1.07)
50–64	16 799	7.2 (6.6, 7.8)	1.19 (1.11, 1.28)	11 806	4.0 (3.5, 4.6)	1.05 (0.94, 1.18)
≥ 65	13 304	7.3 (6.6, 8.0)	1.21 (1.12, 1.31)	9 458	3.2 (2.7, 3.8)	0.86 (0.73, 1.00)
Nationality						
Spanish	65 173	6.0 (5.7, 6.4)	1.00 (0.98, 1.01)	43 084	3.7 (3.4, 4.0)	0.98 (0.96, 0.99)
Other	3 066	6.6 (5.3, 8.2)	1.10 (0.89, 1.34)	1 364	6.4 (4.7, 8.6)	1.69 (1.26, 2.26)
Education[f]						
Less than primary	3 680	6.4 (5.4, 7.6)	0.98 (0.83, 1.15)	2 464	3.7 (2.6, 5.1)	0.98 (0.72, 1.34)
Primary	7 813	6.5 (5.8, 7.4)	0.99 (0.89, 1.11)	5 429	3.5 (2.9, 4.4)	0.95 (0.79, 1.14)
Secondary	14 247	5.8 (5.2, 6.4)	0.88 (0.81, 0.96)	9 724	3.8 (3.3, 4.4)	1.02 (0.90, 1.14)
High school	11 292	7.0 (6.3, 7.7)	1.06 (0.98, 1.15)	7 338	4.4 (3.8, 5.2)	1.19 (1.05, 1.35)
Vocational training	6 369	5.9 (5.2, 6.7)	0.90 (0.79, 1.02)	4 413	3.4 (2.8, 4.1)	0.90 (0.75, 1.09)
University	12 593	7.4 (6.6, 8.2)	1.12 (1.03, 1.22)	8 379	3.4 (2.9, 4.0)	0.91 (0.79, 1.05)
Occupation[f]						
Active worker	28 991	6.9 (6.5, 7.4)	1.07 (1.03, 1.11)	18 186	4.0 (3.6, 4.5)	1.06 (0.99, 1.13)
Unemployed	4 479	4.4 (3.6, 5.4)	0.68 (0.56, 0.82)	3 623	4.1 (3.3, 4.9)	1.07 (0.89, 1.30)
Student	4 230	4.8 (4.0, 5.8)	0.75 (0.63, 0.88)	2 243	4.5 (3.5, 5.8)	1.19 (0.94, 1.49)
Retired	13 239	7.3 (6.6, 8.0)	1.12 (1.04, 1.21)	9 859	3.1 (2.6, 3.7)	0.82 (0.71, 0.95)
Sick leave	1 480	5.5 (4.0, 7.3)	0.84 (0.63, 1.13)	1 163	2.9 (2.0, 4.3)	0.78 (0.54, 1.12)
Homemaker	3 682	5.3 (4.4, 6.3)	0.81 (0.68, 0.96)	2 464	3.9 (3.0, 5.2)	1.04 (0.79, 1.36)
Other	1 017	4.7 (3.3, 6.5)	0.72 (0.52, 1.00)	586	4.4 (2.5, 7.7)	1.16 (0.66, 2.04)
Occupation sector[g]						
Telecommuting	13 159	7.5 (6.9, 8.1)	1.08 (1.02, 1.13)	1 504	3.8 (2.8, 5.3)	0.96 (0.71, 1.29)
Retail	1 869	6.3 (4.9, 8.2)	0.91 (0.72, 1.16)	2 462	3.8 (2.9, 4.9)	0.94 (0.74, 1.19)
Transport	890	6.5 (4.6, 9.1)	0.93 (0.67, 1.30)	744	3.6 (2.2, 5.8)	0.90 (0.57, 1.43)
Security	710	6.9 (4.8, 9.8)	0.99 (0.69, 1.41)	487	5.5 (3.4, 8.8)	1.38 (0.87, 2.19)
Cleaning	902	5.4 (3.7, 7.7)	0.77 (0.54, 1.10)	838	4.9 (3.2, 7.5)	1.22 (0.81, 1.86)
Health care	1 300	11.1 (9.0, 13.6)	1.60 (1.30, 1.95)	990	6.1 (4.4, 8.5)	1.52 (1.10, 2.10)
Nursing home	1 148	10.2 (8.0, 12.8)	1.46 (1.17, 1.82)	831	3.6 (2.2, 5.8)	0.90 (0.56, 1.43)
Home caregiver	454	7.3 (4.4, 11.9)	1.04 (0.64, 1.71)	282	6.0 (3.4, 10.4)	1.50 (0.85, 2.63)
Other	8 457	5.2 (4.6, 5.9)	0.75 (0.68, 0.84)	10 043	3.8 (3.3, 4.3)	0.94 (0.86, 1.03)

Continued

AJPH May 2023, Vol 113, No. 5

TABLE 1— Continued

Characteristic	First Pandemic Wave: No. of Participants[a]	First Pandemic Wave: Seropositivity,[b] % (95% CI)	First Pandemic Wave: Seropositivity Ratio[c] (95% CI)	Second Pandemic Wave: No. of Participants[d]	Second Pandemic Wave: Seropositivity,[e] % (95% CI)	Second Pandemic Wave: Seropositivity Ratio[c] (95% CI)
Smoker[f]						
No	41 881	7.2 (6.7, 7.6)	1.11 (1.08, 1.13)	27 660	4.1 (3.7, 4.5)	1.08 (1.04, 1.12)
Yes	15 885	4.7 (4.2, 5.2)	0.72 (0.66, 0.79)	10 391	3.0 (2.5, 3.5)	0.78 (0.68, 0.98)
Body mass index[f]						
< 25	24 935	6.1 (5.6, 6.6)	0.95 (0.90, 1.00)	15 811	3.6 (3.2, 4.0)	0.94 (0.87, 1.02)
25–29	21 786	6.7 (6.2, 7.2)	1.04 (0.99, 1.09)	14 723	3.8 (3.4, 4.3)	1.01 (0.93, 1.09)
≥ 30	11 164	6.8 (6.1, 7.6)	1.05 (0.96, 1.16)	7 589	4.2 (3.6, 4.9)	1.11 (0.99, 1.25)
No. chronic conditions[h]						
0	21 054	6.9 (6.4, 7.4)	0.97 (0.93, 1.02)	14 093	3.6 (3.2, 4.1)	1.02 (0.94, 1.10)
1	10 338	6.7 (6.1, 7.5)	0.96 (0.88, 1.04)	7 348	3.6 (3.0, 4.2)	1.00 (0.88, 1.15)
2	6 060	8.2 (7.3, 9.2)	1.16 (1.04, 1.30)	4 290	3.4 (2.7, 4.1)	0.94 (0.78, 1.13)
≥ 3	4 318	7.1 (6.1, 8.2)	1.01 (0.88, 1.15)	3 201	3.6 (2.7, 4.7)	0.99 (0.77, 1.28)
Chronic condition[h]						
Diabetes	4 846	6.7 (5.8, 7.8)	0.96 (0.84, 1.09)	3 366	3.2 (2.5, 4.1)	0.90 (0.72, 1.14)
Hypertension	12 145	7.6 (6.9, 8.3)	1.07 (1.00, 1.15)	8 565	3.6 (3.0, 4.2)	1.00 (0.88, 1.13)
CVD	6 034	7.2 (6.3, 8.1)	1.02 (0.91, 1.14)	4 198	3.2 (2.5, 4.1)	0.90 (0.72, 1.12)
Cancer	1 958	7.8 (6.4, 9.5)	1.11 (0.92, 1.34)	1 344	2.6 (1.8, 3.9)	0.73 (0.50, 1.07)
COPD	3 378	7.1 (6.0, 8.2)	1.00 (0.86, 1.16)	2 309	3.5 (2.6, 4.6)	0.97 (0.74, 1.27)
Asthma	2 907	7.7 (6.5, 9.0)	1.07 (0.91, 1.26)	2 205	4.0 (3.0, 5.2)	1.11 (0.86, 1.43)
Sleep apnea	2 277	8.0 (6.6, 9.6)	1.12 (0.94, 1.34)	1 790	4.2 (3.1, 5.6)	1.16 (0.89, 1.53)
CKD	1 352	8.1 (6.4, 10.2)	1.13 (0.90, 1.42)	1 054	3.5 (2.3, 5.2)	0.97 (0.65, 1.44)
IST	1 208	7.5 (5.9, 9.6)	1.05 (0.83, 1.33)	952	3.9 (2.6, 6.0)	1.10 (0.74, 1.64)
CLD	510	6.2 (4.0, 9.6)	0.86 (0.56, 1.31)	475	2.8 (1.5, 5.4)	0.80 (0.42, 1.49)
ACTD	1 118	10.0 (7.8, 12.7)	1.37 (1.08, 1.73)	1 031	3.7 (2.2, 5.9)	1.02 (0.63, 1.65)
Disability, %						
No	62 631	6.1 (5.8, 6.5)	1.00 (0.99, 1.01)	41 718	3.7 (3.4, 4.1)	1.00 (0.99, 1.02)
< 33	583	5.4 (3.5, 8.1)	0.87 (0.57, 1.33)	416	3.0 (1.7, 5.2)	0.79 (0.45, 1.40)
33–65	1 779	6.3 (5.0, 7.9)	1.03 (0.82, 1.28)	1 250	3.8 (2.6, 5.5)	1.01 (0.70, 1.46)
≥ 66	946	5.9 (4.2, 8.2)	0.96 (0.69, 1.33)	650	3.9 (2.1, 7.3)	1.05 (0.57, 1.92)
Household size, no. residents						
1	5 542	6.4 (5.6, 7.3)	1.06 (0.94, 1.19)	2 838	2.6 (2.0, 3.3)	0.68 (0.52, 0.88)
2	15 794	6.9 (6.3, 7.6)	1.15 (1.06, 1.24)	11 295	3.3 (2.8, 3.8)	0.87 (0.75, 1.00)
3–5	43 180	5.8 (5.4, 6.2)	0.95 (0.92, 0.99)	28 021	4.1 (3.7, 4.6)	1.09 (1.04, 1.15)
≥ 6	3 771	4.9 (3.8, 6.3)	0.82 (0.64, 1.04)	2 297	3.3 (2.3, 4.9)	0.88 (0.60, 1.28)
Census tract income, percentile						
< 5th	3 267	5.8 (4.1, 8.2)	0.96 (0.69, 1.36)	1 957	5.4 (3.9, 7.4)	1.43 (1.05, 1.95)
5th–24th	14 915	6.1 (5.3, 7.0)	1.01 (0.88, 1.15)	9 699	4.0 (3.2, 4.9)	1.05 (0.88, 1.27)
25th–49th	17 261	5.9 (5.2, 6.8)	0.98 (0.87, 1.12)	11 173	3.7 (3.2, 4.4)	0.99 (0.85, 1.15)
50th–74th	15 642	5.7 (5.0, 6.6)	0.95 (0.84, 1.08)	10 280	3.9 (3.3, 4.7)	1.03 (0.89, 1.20)
75–94th	13 587	6.2 (5.4, 7.1)	1.02 (0.90, 1.17)	9 146	3.5 (2.8, 4.2)	0.92 (0.77, 1.11)
≥ 95th	3 615	7.4 (5.8, 9.3)	1.22 (0.96, 1.54)	2 196	2.4 (1.6, 3.6)	0.63 (0.42, 0.96)
Municipality size, no. inhabitants						
< 5000	12 167	5.3 (4.6, 6.1)	0.87 (0.76, 1.00)	8 373	4.6 (3.7, 5.8)	1.23 (0.99, 1.52)
5000–19 999	14 439	4.7 (4.1, 5.3)	0.77 (0.68, 0.87)	9 565	3.4 (2.7, 4.3)	0.90 (0.73, 1.11)

Continued

TABLE 1— Continued

Characteristic	First Pandemic Wave			Second Pandemic Wave		
	No. of Participants[a]	Seropositivity,[b] % (95% CI)	Seropositivity Ratio[c] (95% CI)	No. of Participants[d]	Seropositivity,[e] % (95% CI)	Seropositivity Ratio[c] (95% CI)
20 000–99 999	20 652	4.9 (4.4, 5.4)	0.81 (0.74, 0.89)	13 189	3.4 (2.8, 4.0)	0.90 (0.77, 1.04)
≥ 100 000	21 029	7.7 (7.1, 8.4)	1.28 (1.21, 1.35)	13 324	4.0 (3.5, 4.6)	1.05 (0.95, 1.17)

Note. ACTD = autoimmune connective tissue disease; CI = confidence interval; CKD = chronic kidney disease; CLD = chronic liver disease; COPD = chronic obstructive pulmonary disease; CVD = cardiovascular disease; ENE-COVID = Spanish National Seroepidemiological Survey of SARS-CoV-2 Infection/Estudio Nacional de Sero-Epidemiología de la Infección por SARS-CoV-2 en España; IST = immunosuppressive therapy; SARS-CoV-2 = severe acute respiratory syndrome coronavirus 2.

[a]Participants who received the point-of-care test in at least 1 of the 3 rounds of the first survey phase.
[b]Proportion of participants who had detectable immunoglobulin G antibodies against SARS-CoV-2 in any round of the first survey phase by the point-of-care test.
[c]Seropositivity ratio with respect to all combined categories of a given characteristic.
[d]Participants who tested negative by all received point-of-care tests during the first phase and underwent the test in the single round of the second survey phase.
[e]Proportion of seronegative participants in the first phase who had detectable immunoglobulin G antibodies against SARS-CoV-2 in the single round of the second survey phase by the point-of-care test.
[f]Among participants aged 17 y or older. Body mass index is defined as weight in kilograms divided by the square of height in meters.
[g]Among active workers.
[h]Among participants aged 40 y or older. Number of chronic conditions computed from those listed in the table.

AJPH May 2023, Vol 113, No. 5

and women). During the first pandemic wave, 6.0% of the Spanish population became infected. There were striking geographical differences (Figure 1), with seroprevalences greater than 10% concentrated in the middle of the country, whereas most of the coastal provinces had values lower than 4%. Table 1 shows seroprevalence figures and seroprevalence ratios according to different sociodemographic characteristics. Global prevalence figures were similar in both genders.

Seropositivity increased with age, being lower among those younger than 20 years (4%) and higher in those 50 years and older (7%). This pattern was observed in both males and females (Figure 2), although seroprevalence peaked at approximately 75 years in women only. As seen in Table 1, prevalence of infection was higher in people with a bachelor's degree or higher (SPR = 1.12; 95% CI = 1.03, 1.22), particularly among men (Table A), those living in census tracts with higher income (SPR = 1.22; 95% CI = 0.96, 1.54), and those living in cities (SPR = 1.28; 95% CI = 1.21, 1.35). Health care and nursing home workers were more affected than were workers in other occupational sectors with activity during the lockdown (SPR = 1.60; 95% CI = 1.30, 1.95 and SPR = 1.46; 95% CI = 1.17, 1.82, respectively). Smokers had lower seroprevalence than did nonsmokers (4.7% vs 7.2%).

During the second wave, 3.8% of participants were newly seropositive. The geographical distribution was more diffuse (Figure 1). Highest de novo seroprevalences were observed in northeast Spain, whereas the middle of the country was still more affected. Again, no differences were observed by gender, but the age distribution was different in men and women (Figure 2). The highest seroprevalence was observed in those aged 20 to 29 years and in men, with a clear downward trend after aged 75 years. This trend was not as clear in females, who had a constant percentage of new seropositive participants from children aged 5 to 9 years to adults aged 80 to 84 years. In this pandemic wave, Spanish participants were less affected than were those from other countries (3.7 vs 6.4%; Table 1), with no differences between men and women (Table A).

Those who worked in the security (SPR = 1.38; 95% CI = 0.87, 2.19), cleaning (SPR = 1.22; 95% CI = 0.81, 1.86), health care (SPR = 1.52; 95% CI = 1.10, 2.10), and home care (SPR = 1.50; 95% CI = 0.85, 2.63) sectors had higher seropositivity, whereas nursing home workers were not among those more affected (SPR = 0.90; 95% CI = 0.56, 1.43). The analysis by gender showed high risk in security workers among men, cleaners and nursing home workers among women, and health care workers among both genders (Table A). Unlike what was observed in the first wave, the most affected areas were low-income census tracts (SPR = 1.43; 95% CI = 1.05, 1.95) and smaller towns

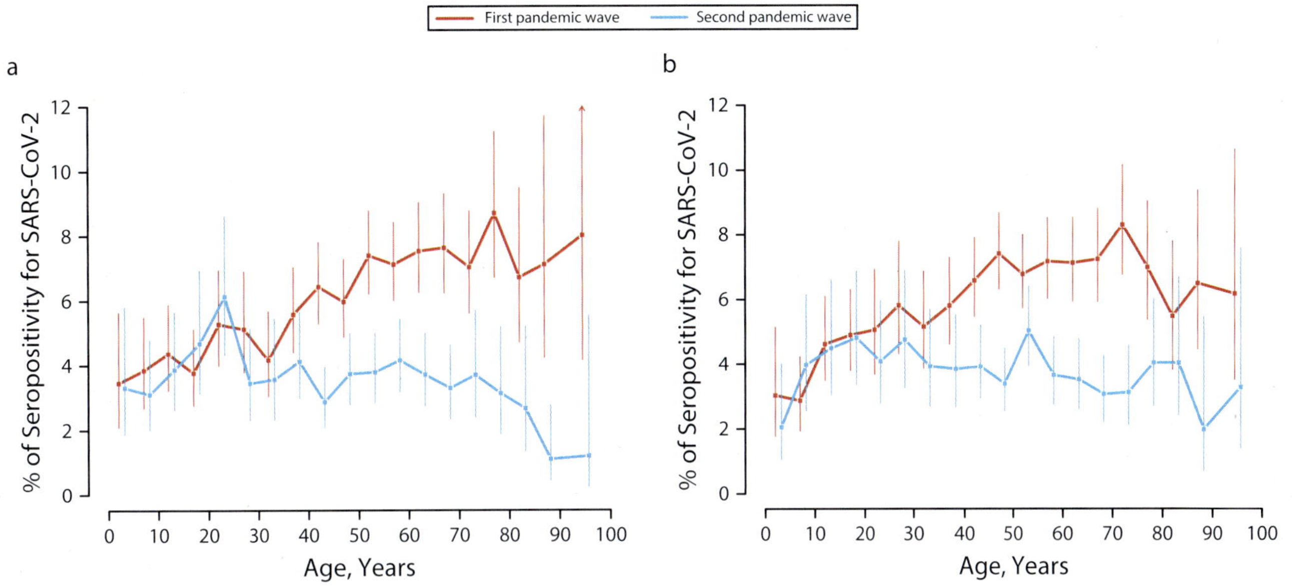

FIGURE 2— New Seropositive Participants for SARS-CoV-2 as Determined by the Point-of-Care Test in the First and Second Pandemic Waves by Age Among (a) Men and (b) Women: ENE-COVID, Spain, April 27–June 22 and November 16–30, 2020

Note. ENE-COVID = Spanish National Seroepidemiological Survey of SARS-CoV-2 Infection/Estudio Nacional de Sero-Epidemiología de la Infección por SARS-CoV-2 en España; SARS-CoV-2 = severe acute respiratory syndrome coronavirus 2. Vertical lines represent 95% confidence intervals.

(SPR = 1.23; 95% CI = 0.99, 1.52). Finally, de novo seropositivity was also lower among smokers than those who did not smoke (3.0% vs 4.1%).

Table 2 presents the same figures according to COVID-19–related factors. As expected, in both waves symptoms and antecedents of a positive PCR result were strongly associated with a positive serological result (SPR > 2). Every type of contact with those with confirmed or suspected COVID-19 increased the risk, but estimates were highest if the contact was with household members, especially in the second pandemic wave (SPR = 3.65 and 9.25 during the first and second waves, respectively, for cohabitant with confirmed COVID-19; SPR = 2.46 and 6.97 for cohabitant suspected to have COVID-19 in the corresponding wave). Analyses by gender did not show remarkable differences in the influence of these factors (Appendix Table B).

Seropositivity determined by the CMIA decreased to 4.9% and 3.3% during the first and second pandemic waves, respectively. Results were like those for the point-of-care test, although estimates were less precise because the CMIA was offered to only a random subcohort in the second wave (Appendix Tables C and D). In sensitivity analyses combining both tests, seropositivity ranged from 3.9% (95% CI = 3.6%, 4.2% when both tests were positive) to 7.3% (95% CI = 6.9%, 7.7% when either test was positive) in the first wave and from 2.6% (95% CI = 1.9%, 3.4%) to 4.3% (95% CI = 3.5%, 5.3%) in the second wave. Second to first wave seropositivity ratios were 0.65 (95% CI = 0.48, 0.89) for both tests positive and 0.58 (95% CI = 0.47, 0.72) for either test positive, which were like ratios obtained for each test separately: 0.63 (95% CI = 0.56, 0.70) for the point-of-care test and 0.68 (95% CI = 0.52, 0.89) for the CMIA.

DISCUSSION

According to ENE-COVID, between 5% and 6% of the noninstitutionalized population had been infected by SARS-CoV-2 by June 2020 in Spain, during the first pandemic wave, which suggests 2.3 to 2.8 million people were infected. To these figures, we should add those occurring in nursing homes, not included in the ENE-COVID design, which were heavily affected.[5] Our results suggest that, at that moment, fewer than 1 in 10 infections were diagnosed and registered in the RENAVE (the National Epidemiological Surveillance System).[6] There was a severe shortage of PCR tests, which were reserved for hospitalized patients and for symptomatic essential workers, mainly health care professionals—a sector with a clear predominance of women (74%).[7] This created a distorted picture of the situation, with more than 40% of notified

AJPH May 2023, Vol 113, No. 5

TABLE 2— New Seropositive Participants for SARS-CoV-2 as Determined by the Point-of-Care Test in the First and Second Pandemic Waves by COVID-19–Related Characteristics: ENE–COVID, Spain, April 27–June 22 and November 16–30, 2020

	First Pandemic Wave			Second Pandemic Wave		
Characteristic[a]	No. of Participants[b]	Seropositivity,[c] % (95% CI)	Seropositivity Ratio[d] (95% CI)	No. of Participants[e]	Seropositivity,[f] % (95% CI)	Seropositivity Ratio[d] (95% CI)
Symptoms compatible with COVID-19[g]						
Asymptomatic	42 275	3.7 (3.4, 3.9)	0.61 (0.57, 0.64)	35 674	1.8 (1.6, 2.1)	0.48 (0.44, 0.53)
Paucisymptomatic	15 663	5.1 (4.6, 5.6)	0.84 (0.77, 0.91)	5 715	5.1 (4.3, 6.0)	1.34 (1.17, 1.53)
Symptomatic	10 346	16.5 (15.3, 17.8)	2.73 (2.59, 2.87)	3 062	22.3 (20.0, 24.7)	5.90 (5.45, 6.38)
Time since symptom onset, d						
≤ 14	362	15.2 (10.9, 20.8)	2.51 (1.83, 3.46)	420	8.3 (5.5, 12.5)	2.21 (1.46, 3.33)
> 14[h]	9 984	16.5 (15.3, 17.8)	2.73 (2.60, 2.88)	2 642	24.6 (22.1, 27.4)	6.53 (6.01, 7.08)
PCR status						
Never tested	62 198	5.9 (5.5, 6.2)	0.97 (0.96, 0.99)	34 365	1.8 (1.6, 2.0)	0.47 (0.42, 0.51)
Negative	5 538	3.4 (2.8, 4.1)	0.56 (0.47, 0.67)	8 749	3.0 (2.5, 3.6)	0.80 (0.68, 0.94)
Positive ≤ 14 d	33	58.5 (34.0, 79.4)	9.68 (6.38, 14.7)	100	47.1 (34.7, 59.9)	12.47 (9.49, 16.4)
Positive > 14 d[h]	353	66.4 (58.6, 73.4)	10.99 (9.82, 12.3)	1 192	64.1 (59.9, 68.0)	16.96 (15.6, 18.4)
Awaiting result	161	9.3 (4.6, 17.8)	1.53 (0.78, 3.03)	44	0.9 (0.2, 4.4)	0.25 (0.05, 1.19)
Contact with confirmed case						
No contact	60 591	5.0 (4.7, 5.3)	0.83 (0.80, 0.85)	36 519	1.9 (1.7, 2.2)	0.51 (0.47, 0.56)
Household member	1 897	22.1 (18.9, 25.6)	3.65 (3.15, 4.24)	1 424	35.0 (30.8, 39.4)	9.25 (8.30, 10.3)
Noncohabitating family/friend	2 518	10.6 (9.1, 12.4)	1.76 (1.52, 2.03)	3 145	11.1 (9.3, 13.2)	2.94 (2.55, 3.38)
Co-worker	2 169	10.9 (9.1, 13.0)	1.80 (1.52, 2.13)	1 916	5.3 (4.2, 6.7)	1.41 (1.14, 1.75)
Cleaning person/caregiver	127	11.7 (6.4, 20.6)	1.94 (1.07, 3.52)	102	11.6 (4.9, 25.1)	3.07 (1.35, 7.02)
Patient/client	1 437	10.8 (8.8, 13.1)	1.78 (1.47, 2.16)	755	6.5 (4.5, 9.3)	1.72 (1.19, 2.48)
Classmate	N/A	N/A	N/A	1 033	4.8 (3.3, 6.9)	1.27 (0.90, 1.80)
Contact with symptomatic person						
No contact	55 507	4.3 (4.0, 4.6)	0.71 (0.68, 0.74)	40 182	2.8 (2.5, 3.1)	0.74 (0.70, 0.78)
Household member	5 465	14.9 (13.3, 16.6)	2.46 (2.24, 2.70)	1 083	26.3 (22.3, 30.8)	6.97 (5.96, 8.15)
Noncohabitating family/friend	3 215	11.7 (10.1, 13.5)	1.93 (1.70, 2.20)	1 377	12.4 (9.9, 15.5)	3.29 (2.69, 4.04)
Co-worker	2 991	11.0 (9.5, 12.7)	1.82 (1.59, 2.08)	945	6.7 (4.9, 8.9)	1.76 (1.33, 2.34)
Cleaning person/caregiver	167	6.6 (3.4, 12.2)	1.09 (0.57, 2.07)	36	5.4 (1.7, 16.2)	1.44 (0.46, 4.55)
Patient/client	1 499	10.1 (8.2, 12.4)	1.67 (1.37, 2.05)	544	8.2 (5.4, 12.4)	2.18 (1.44, 3.29)
Classmate	N/A	N/A	N/A	470	4.7 (2.9, 7.8)	1.26 (0.76, 2.07)

Note. CI = confidence interval; ENE–COVID = Spanish National Seroepidemiological Survey of SARS-CoV-2 Infection/Estudio Nacional de Sero-Epidemiología de la Infección por SARS-CoV-2 en España; N/A = not available; PCR = polymerase chain reaction; SARS-CoV-2 = severe acute respiratory syndrome coronavirus 2.

[a]For the first pandemic wave, information up to the last round of participation of the first survey phase or the first round with positive result as determined by the point-of-care test; for the second pandemic wave, information after the end of the first wave (July 1, 2020).
[b]Participants who received the point-of-care test in at least 1 of the 3 rounds of the first survey phase.
[c]Proportion of participants who had detectable immunoglobulin G antibodies against SARS-CoV-2 in any round of the first survey phase as determined by the point-of-care test.
[d]Seropositivity ratio with respect to all combined categories of a given characteristic.
[e]Participants who tested negative by all received point-of-care tests during the first phase and underwent the test in the single round of the second survey phase.
[f]Proportion of seronegative participants in the first phase who had detectable immunoglobulin G antibodies against SARS-CoV-2 in the single round of the second survey phase as determined by the point-of-care test.
[g]Asymptomatic (no symptoms), paucisymptomatic (1–2 symptoms without anosmia/ageusia), and symptomatic (anosmia/ageusia or at least 3 symptoms among fever, chills, severe tiredness, sore throat, cough, shortness of breath, headache, and nausea/vomiting/diarrhea).
[h]For the first pandemic wave > 14 d before any round of participation of the first survey phase or before the first round with positive result as determined by the point-of-care test.

infected individuals among people 70 years and older and a predominance of women over men.[1]

By contrast, the first 3 rounds of ENE–COVID showed similar seroprevalences in males and females, whereas the differences by age were much attenuated. Regarding the geographical distribution, ENE–COVID confirmed the higher prevalence in Madrid, Castilla-La Mancha, and Castilla y León (the center of the country) and Barcelona (in the northeast). Navarre and La Rioja were hotspots according to the RENAVE data,[1] but they did not have very high seroprevalence figures. This discordance suggests differences in the availability of diagnostic tests across Spanish autonomous communities.

The first pandemic wave in Spain was dominated by 2 early clades closely related to Asian SARS-CoV-2 variants.[8,9] The outbreak overwhelmed the health care system in several Spanish regions.[10] Health care workers were overstressed and insufficiently protected[11,12] and, according to our results, 1 in 10 was infected during this period. The national lockdown, enforced at the peak of the pandemic, included school closure, workplace closure, and mobility restrictions and served to reverse the trend and contain the viral transmission.[9,13] At the end of June 2020, the country slowly recovered mobility and economic activity, although some restrictions were maintained, including the mandatory use of face masks. A new variant, B.1.177 (initially named 20E.EU1), with increased transmissibility was identified early that summer in the country and later became dominant in Europe.[14]

The second pandemic wave started to escalate in July to August 2020, and the Spanish government declared a second state of emergency at the peak of the second wave, October 25, but did not impose a national lockdown. In this case, autonomous communities implemented different public health interventions over time. By the middle of November, when the last round of ENE–COVID started, there were more than 1 million new cases reported to the RENAVE, many of them asymptomatic.[6] However, according to ENE–COVID estimates, between 3.3% and 3.8% of house-dwelling people were newly infected by SARS-CoV-2, that is, approximately 1.5 to 1.6 million people. The highest de novo seropositivity was observed in the northeast of the country.

Again, men and women were equally affected, but the age distribution was different during the second wave. Among previously uninfected men, the highest seroprevalence occurred at age 20 to 29 years, and the oldest age groups had the lowest risk. In women, the distribution was somehow more homogeneous, but lowest rates were also observed among older women. These disparities correlate well with the reported differences in risk perception toward COVID-19 by age and gender in Spain,[15] suggesting that older people, particularly men, stayed at home more often and tended to avoid social contact,[4] reducing their infection risk.[16] In women, differences were less obvious, and although they have been reported to be more cautious,[15] their role at home and as caregivers may have presented more opportunities to become infected.[17]

Big cities, with greater international exchange and greater population density, had a higher seroprevalence during the first wave. However, the pandemic moved from the cities to the rural areas during the summer, with smaller municipalities having the highest seroprevalence in the second wave. Restrictions on traveling outside Spain, together with increased concern about becoming infected abroad, made people spend their summer holidays inside the country, choosing less populated places.

The ENE–COVID study was not designed to explore socioeconomic differences in detail, but some individual and ecological information allowed us to explore this aspect. Highly educated men and people living in wealthier census tracts were more frequently infected at the beginning of the pandemic, possibly because of their greater international mobility.[9] The first pandemic wave took everybody by surprise, and even though some reports found stronger effects in areas with lower socioeconomic status within big cities, such as Barcelona,[18] the national lockdown seemed to attenuate them. Later, as the virus was widely disseminated, disadvantaged socioeconomic groups were at higher risk of infection. During the second pandemic wave, participants living in lower income census tracts and non-Spanish people were more affected. These socioeconomic differences have been observed in other countries,[19–23] and a combination of factors, related to work and home conditions, may explain them.[24,25] In fact, the first big outbreaks that summer occurred in occupational settings,[26] and, as ENE–COVID shows, essential low-wage occupations, such as cleaners and home caregivers, were at higher risk for infection.

Living with someone who was confirmed or suspected to be infected was the strongest risk factor for being seropositive, especially in the second wave, reflecting the difficulty of isolating those infected with SARS-CoV-2 at home. Even though some autonomous communities provided specific places to isolate infected people if needed (e.g., hotels), these resources were not generally available. Also, in the second wave, risk of infection was higher after contact with friends or noncohabiting relatives who were confirmed or suspected to be infected than after contact at work, suggesting lower success of public health measures in informal settings.

Of note, in both waves, smokers had lower seroprevalence values. It is unlikely that this result is attributable to selection bias, and our data support studies that suggest smokers have a reduced risk of infection.[27]

Strengths and Limitations

This study updates the epidemiological information on the first pandemic wave in Spain. It considered 3 consecutive survey rounds and describes for the first time, to our knowledge, the characteristics of the second pandemic wave. With a population-based design and high percentages of participation, ENE–COVID provided an accurate representation of the situation of SARS-CoV-2 infection in the whole country. In this sense, our random selection sampling design, as well as our use of poststratification sampling weights, which served to correct regional income, age, and gender differences in participation, are 2 of the strongest points of ENE–COVID. The National Centre for Microbiology of the Instituto de Salud Carlos III selected the serological tests after carefully screening those available.

ENE–COVID also has several limitations. It did not study the situation of institutionalized people, as they required a different approach. Although only 6% of participants older than 75 years reside in nursing homes,[28] they suffered many outbreaks with very high mortality.[4,5] Also, the information relies on detection of anti-SARS-CoV-2 IgG antibodies, which appear 1 to 3 weeks after infection.[29] Apart from the false positive and negative results associated with the characteristics of the test, a low proportion of infected people, particularly those who are asymptomatic, do not seroconvert,[29,30] whereas those who become positive may test negative after several months.[29] Seroreversion, however, is not an issue here, because ENE–COVID started at the end of April, just a month after the peak of the first pandemic wave.

Finally, the second pandemic wave was still trending downward when the study took place, leading us to underestimate new seroprevalence figures. Also, this last round of the survey had lower participation, possibly because of a loss of interest in being tested given the greater availability of diagnostic and serological tools. Still, almost 7 of 10 participants who were previously seronegative agreed to participate. Results for this wave are based mainly on the point-of-care test, because venipuncture was offered only to a subsample of seronegative participants to facilitate the fieldwork in primary health centers, which were still severely overloaded because of the pandemic.[31]

Conclusions

ENE–COVID served to characterize the first 2 pandemic waves of SARS-CoV-2 and provided useful information when data on COVID-19 cases and new infections were insufficient. People living in the center of Spain, those living in cities, and those with higher education were more affected during the first wave. However, the virus spread across the country, particularly toward the northeast, and more disadvantaged groups were at higher risk for infection after lifting the national lockdown. Health workers and individuals in other occupations who take care of vulnerable people suffered higher rates of infection. In both waves, living with someone who had COVID-19 strongly influenced the probability of being infected.

Public Health Implications

From a public health surveillance standpoint, ENE–COVID has provided health authorities key and timely information on the COVID-19 pandemic as follows:

- Seroprevalence studies are useful for providing information when there is incomplete case ascertainment and there may be a substantial proportion of asymptomatic infections.
- Contrary to the picture drawn by the National Epidemiological Surveillance System, we learned that the virus infected men and women equally and that all age groups were at risk.
- According to seroprevalence figures, the proportion of people infected during these 2 pandemic waves was insufficient to guarantee herd immunity.
- Health care workers suffered the brunt of the new pandemic, with seroprevalence figures that were almost double those found in the overall population.
- Living with an infected person was the strongest avoidable risk factor; public health strategies should give households more attention.
- Older people, who were at higher risk of death, had a lower relative infection rate in the second wave.
- Socioeconomic differences appeared during the second wave.

In situations like this, specific measures are needed to protect disadvantaged groups.

It is important to highlight the added value of the longitudinal design of ENE–COVID, which allowed us to explore changes in the epidemiological characteristics of the pandemic over time. AJPH

ABOUT THE AUTHORS

Beatriz Pérez-Gómez, Roberto Pastor-Barriuso, Nerea Fernández-de-Larrea, Pablo Fernández-Navarro, and Marina Pollán are with the National Centre for Epidemiology and the Consortium for Biomedical Research in Epidemiology and Public Health (CIBERESP), Instituto de Salud Carlos III (ISCIII), Madrid, Spain. Miguel A. Hernán is with the Departments of Epidemiology and Biostatistics, Harvard T. H. Chan School of Public Health, Boston, MA. Mayte Pérez-Olmeda, Jesús Oteo-Iglesias, and Aurora Fernández-García are with the National Centre for Microbiology and the Consortium for Biomedical Research in Infectious Diseases (CIBERINFEC), ISCIII. Mariano Martín, José L. Sanmartín, Juan F. Muñoz-Montalvo, and Faustino Blanco are with the Deputy Directorate of Information Technologies, Ministry of Health, Madrid, Spain. Israel Cruz is with the National School of Public Health, ISCIII. José León-Paniagua and Raquel Yotti are with ISCIII.

CORRESPONDENCE

Correspondence should be sent to Marina Pollán, National Centre for Epidemiology, Instituto de Salud Carlos III, Monforte de Lemos 5, 28029 Madrid, Spain (e-mail: mpollan@isciii.es). Reprints can be ordered at http://www.ajph.org by clicking the "Reprints" link.

PUBLICATION INFORMATION

Full Citation: Pérez-Gómez B, Pastor-Barriuso R, Fernández-de-Larrea N, et al. SARS-CoV-2 infection during the first and second pandemic waves in Spain: the ENE–COVID study. *Am J Public Health*. 2023;113(5):533–544.

Acceptance Date: January 7, 2023.

DOI: https://doi.org/10.2105/AJPH.2023.307233

CONTRIBUTORS

B. Pérez-Gómez, R. Pastor-Barriuso, and N. Fernández-de-Larrea contributed equally to the article. B. Pérez-Gómez, R. Pastor-Barriuso, and M. Pollán were responsible for the conceptualization and design of the study. B. Pérez-Gómez, R. Pastor-Barriuso, N. Fernández-de-Larrea, M. A. Hernán, P. Fernández-Navarro, and M. Pollán led analyses and table and figure design. B. Pérez-Gómez, R. Pastor-Barriuso, and M. Pollán drafted the article, and the remaining authors provided significant input, review, and editing. M. Pérez-Olmeda, J. Oteo-Iglesias, and A. Fernández-García were responsible for the validation of serological tests, coordination of microbiological laboratories, and acquisition of laboratory data. M. Martín, J. L. Sanmartín, J. León-Paniagua, and J. F. Muñoz-Montalvo were responsible for the study operation, including the coordination of data acquisition and logistics. I. Cruz developed the operational protocols for fieldwork and was responsible for training administrative and health personnel. F. Blanco and R. Yotti were the executive coordinators of the project and led the relationship with regional health services. All authors read and approved the final version of the article.

ACKNOWLEDGMENTS

This work was supported by the Spanish Ministry of Health, the Institute of Health Carlos III (Ministry of Science and Innovation), and the National Health System, including the Health Services of all autonomous communities and autonomous cities: Servicio Andaluz de Salud, Servicio Aragonés de Salud, Servicio de Salud del Principado de Asturias, Servei de Salut Illes Balears, Servicio Canario de la Salud, Servicio Cántabro de Salud, Servicio de Salud de Castilla-La Mancha, Servicio de Salud de Castilla y León, Servei Català de Salut, Conselleria de Sanitat Universal i Salut Pública de la Generalitat Valenciana, Servicio Extremeño de Salud, Servizo Galego de Saúde, Servicio Riojano de Salud, Servicio Madrileño de Salud, Servicio Murciano de Salud, Servicio Navarro de Salud-Osasunbidea and Instituto de Salud Pública y Laboral de Navarra, Servicio Vasco de Salud-Osakidetza, and Instituto de Gestión Sanitaria.

We thank all the nurses, general practitioners, administrative personnel, and other health care workers who collaborated in this study and all participants. This study is the result of the efforts of many professionals and the trust and generosity of more than 68 000 participants who understood the importance of providing time, information, and samples to learn about the COVID-19 pandemic in Spain. The Spanish Institute of Statistics provided the random selection of households and the information required to contact participants.

Collaborators of the ENE–COVID Study Group (Spanish National Seroepidemiological Survey of SARS-CoV-2 Infection/Estudio Nacional de Sero-Epidemiología de la Infección por SARS-CoV-2 en España) are listed in the Appendix (available as a supplement to the online version of this article at http://www.ajph.org).

CONFLICTS OF INTEREST

M. A. Hernán is a consultant for Cytel and adviser for ProPublica. The other authors have no conflicts of interest to declare.

HUMAN PARTICIPANT PROTECTION

The Institute of Health Carlos III institutional review board (ISCIII Committee for Ethical Research) approved the study (register No. PI 39_2020).

REFERENCES

1. Working Group for the Surveillance and Control of COVID-19 in Spain. The first wave of the COVID-19 pandemic in Spain: characterisation of cases and risk factors for severe outcomes, as at 27 April 2020. *Euro Surveill.* 2020;25(50):2001431. https://doi.org/10.2807/1560-7917.ES.2020.25.50.2001431
2. Pollán M, Pérez-Gómez B, Pastor-Barriuso R, et al. Prevalence of SARS-CoV-2 in Spain (ENE-COVID): a nationwide, population-based seroepidemiological study. *Lancet.* 2020;396(10250):535–544. https://doi.org/10.1016/S0140-6736(20)31483-5
3. Instituto de Salud Carlos III. National Study of SARS-CoV-2 Sero-Epidemiology in Spain (ENE–COVID). 2020. Available at: https://portalcne.isciii.es/enecovid19. Accessed July 29, 2022.
4. Pastor-Barriuso R, Pérez-Gómez B, Hernán MA, et al. Infection fatality risk for SARS-CoV-2 in community dwelling population of Spain: nationwide seroepidemiological study. *BMJ.* 2020;371:m4509. https://doi.org/10.1136/bmj.m4509
5. IMSERSO. Informe Del Grupo de Trabajo COVID 19 y Residencias. 2020. Available at: https://www.imserso.es/InterPresent1/groups/imserso/documents/binario/gtcovid_residencias_vf.pdf. Accessed August 20, 2022.
6. Instituto de Salud Carlos III. COVID-19 in Spain. 2020. Available at: https://cnecovid.isciii.es/covid19. Accessed July 24, 2020.
7. Nova IP. Radiografía del papel de la mujer en la sanidad española. *Redacción Médica*. March 8, 2018. Available at: https://www.redaccionmedica.com/secciones/sanidad-hoy/radiografia-del-papel-de-la-mujer-en-la-sanidad-espanola-1050. Accessed September 19, 2020.
8. Díez-Fuertes F, Iglesias-Caballero M, García-Pérez J, et al. A founder effect led early SARS-CoV-2 transmission in Spain. *J Virol.* 2021;95(3):e01583–e015820. https://doi.org/10.1128/JVI.01583-20
9. López MG, Chiner-Oms Á, García de Viedma D, et al. The first wave of the COVID-19 epidemic in Spain was associated with early introductions and fast spread of a dominating genetic variant. *Nat Genet.* 2021;53(10):1405–1414. https://doi.org/10.1038/s41588-021-00936-6
10. Martínez-Alés G, Domingo-Relloso A, Arribas JR, Quintana-Díaz M, Hernán MA; COVID@HULP Group. Critical care requirements under uncontrolled transmission of SARS-CoV-2. *Am J Public Health.* 2021;111(5):923–926. https://doi.org/10.2105/AJPH.2020.306151
11. Alonso J, Vilagut G, Mortier P, et al. Mental health impact of the first wave of COVID-19 pandemic on Spanish healthcare workers: a large cross-sectional survey. *Rev Psiquiatr Salud Ment (Engl Ed).* 2021;14(2):90–105. https://doi.org/10.1016/j.rpsm.2020.12.001
12. González-Gil MT, González-Blázquez C, Parro-Moreno AI, et al. Nurses' perceptions and demands regarding COVID-19 care delivery in critical care units and hospital emergency services. *Intensive Crit Care Nurs.* 2021;62:102966. https://doi.org/10.1016/j.iccn.2020.102966
13. Islam N, Sharp SJ, Chowell G, et al. Physical distancing interventions and incidence of coronavirus disease 2019: natural experiment in 149 countries. *BMJ.* 2020;370:m2743. https://doi.org/10.1136/bmj.m2743
14. Hodcroft EB, Zuber M, Nadeau S, et al. Spread of a SARS-CoV-2 variant through Europe in the summer

of 2020. *Nature.* 2021;595(7869):707–712. https://doi.org/10.1038/s41586-021-03677-y

15. Recio-Vivas AM, Font-Jiménez I, Mansilla-Domínguez JM, et al. Fear and attitude towards SARS-CoV-2 (COVID-19) infection in Spanish population during the period of confinement. *Int J Environ Res Public Health.* 2022;19(2):834. https://doi.org/10.3390/ijerph19020834
16. Andrasfay T, Wu Q, Lee H, Crimmins EM. Adherence to social-distancing and personal hygiene behavior guidelines and risk of COVID-19 diagnosis: evidence from the Understanding America Study. *Am J Public Health.* 2022;112(1):169–178. https://doi.org/10.2105/AJPH.2021.306565
17. Ayittey FK, Dhar BK, Anani G, Chiwero NB. Gendered burdens and impacts of SARS-CoV-2: a review. *Health Care Women Int.* 2020;41(11–12):1210–1225. https://doi.org/10.1080/07399332.2020.1809664
18. Baena-Díez JM, Barroso M, Cordeiro-Coelho SI, Díaz JL, Grau M. Impact of COVID-19 outbreak by income: hitting hardest the most deprived. *J Public Health (Oxf).* 2020;42(4):698–703. https://doi.org/10.1093/pubmed/fdaa136
19. Plümper T, Neumayer E. The pandemic predominantly hits poor neighbourhoods? SARS-CoV-2 infections and COVID-19 fatalities in German districts. *Eur J Public Health.* 2020;30(6):1176–1180. https://doi.org/10.1093/eurpub/ckaa168
20. Carrat F, de Lamballerie X, Rahib D, et al. Antibody status and cumulative incidence of SARS-CoV-2 infection among adults in three regions of France following the first lockdown and associated risk factors: a multicohort study. *Int J Epidemiol.* 2021;50(5):1458–1472. [Erratum in: *Int J Epidemiol.* Aug 28, 2021]. https://doi.org/10.1093/ije/dyab110
21. Saarinen S, Moustgaard H, Remes H, Sallinen R, Martikainen P. Income differences in COVID-19 incidence and severity in Finland among people with foreign and native background: a population-based cohort study of individuals nested within households. *PLoS Med.* 2022;19(8):e1004038. https://doi.org/10.1371/journal.pmed.1004038
22. Tai DBG, Shah A, Doubeni CA, Sia IG, Wieland ML. The disproportionate impact of COVID-19 on racial and ethnic minorities in the United States. *Clin Infect Dis.* 2021;72(4):703–706. https://doi.org/10.1093/cid/ciaa815
23. Khanijahani A, Iezadi S, Gholipour K, Azami-Aghdash S, Naghibi D. A systematic review of racial/ethnic and socioeconomic disparities in COVID-19. *Int J Equity Health.* 2021;20(1):248. https://doi.org/10.1186/s12939-021-01582-4
24. Burström B, Tao W. Social determinants of health and inequalities in COVID-19. *Eur J Public Health.* 2020;30(4):617–618. https://doi.org/10.1093/eurpub/ckaa095
25. Anderson G, Frank JW, Naylor CD, Wodchis W, Feng P. Using socioeconomics to counter health disparities arising from the COVID-19 pandemic. *BMJ.* 2020;369:m2149. https://doi.org/10.1136/bmj.m2149
26. National COVID-19 Outbreak Monitoring Group. COVID-19 outbreaks in a transmission control scenario: challenges posed by social and leisure activities, and for workers in vulnerable conditions, Spain, early summer 2020. *Euro Surveill.* 2020;25(35):2001545. https://doi.org/10.2807/1560-7917.ES.2020.25.35.2001545
27. Paleiron N, Mayet A, Marbac V, et al. Impact of tobacco smoking on the risk of COVID-19: a large scale retrospective cohort study. *Nicotine Tob Res.* 2021;23(8):1398–1404. https://doi.org/10.1093/ntr/ntab004
28. Abellan García A, Aceituno Nieto P, Fernández Morales I, Ramiro Fariñas D, Pujol Rodríguez R. Una estimación de la población que vive en residencias de mayores—EnR. April 24, 2020. Available at: http://envejecimientoenred.es/una-estimacion-de-la-poblacion-que-vive-en-residencias-de-mayores. Accessed May 22, 2020.
29. Wei J, Matthews PC, Stoesser N, et al. Anti-spike antibody response to natural SARS-CoV-2 infection in the general population. *Nat Commun.* 2021;12(1):6250. https://doi.org/10.1038/s41467-021-26479-2
30. Petersen LR, Sami S, Vuong N, et al. Lack of antibodies to severe acute respiratory syndrome coronavirus 2 (SARS-CoV-2) in a large cohort of previously infected persons. *Clin Infect Dis.* 2021;73(9):e3066–e3073. https://doi.org/10.1093/cid/ciaa1685
31. Fernández-Aguilar C, Casado-Aranda LA, Farrés Fernández M, Minué Lorenzo S. Has COVID-19 changed the workload for primary care physicians? The case of Spain. *Fam Pract.* 2021;38(6):780–785. https://doi.org/10.1093/fampra/cmab028

Design and Implementation of a National SARS-CoV-2 Monitoring Program in England: REACT-1 Study

Paul Elliott, PhD, Matthew Whitaker, MSc, David Tang, MSc, Oliver Eales, PhD, Nicholas Steyn, BSc, Barbara Bodinier, PhD, Haowei Wang, MSc, Joshua Elliott, MSc, Christina Atchison, PhD, Deborah Ashby, PhD, Wendy Barclay, PhD, Graham Taylor, DSc, Ara Darzi, MD, Graham S. Cooke, PhD, Helen Ward, PhD, Christl A. Donnelly, ScD, Steven Riley, DPhil, and Marc Chadeau-Hyam, PhD

See also Morabia, p. 462, Elliott et al., p. 514, Dean et al., p. 517, Jernigan et al., p. 520, Bendavid, p. 523, Pastor-Barriuso et al., p. 525, and Pérez-Gómez et al., p. 533.

Data System. The REal-time Assessment of Community Transmission-1 (REACT-1) Study was funded by the Department of Health and Social Care in England to provide reliable and timely estimates of prevalence of severe acute respiratory syndrome coronavirus 2 (SARS-CoV-2) infection over time, by person and place.

Data Collection/Processing. The study team (researchers from Imperial College London and its logistics partner Ipsos) wrote to named individuals aged 5 years and older in random cross-sections of the population of England, using the National Health Service list of patients registered with a general practitioner (near-universal coverage) as a sampling frame. We collected data over 2 to 3 weeks approximately every month across 19 rounds of data collection from May 1, 2020, to March 31, 2022.

Data Analysis/Dissemination. We have disseminated the data and study materials widely via the study Web site, preprints, publications in peer-reviewed journals, and the media. We make available data tabulations, suitably anonymized to protect participant confidentiality, on request to the study's data access committee.

Public Health Implications. The study provided inter alia real-time data on SARS-CoV-2 prevalence over time, by area, and by sociodemographic variables; estimates of vaccine effectiveness; and symptom profiles, and detected emergence of new variants based on viral genome sequencing. (*Am J Public Health*. 2023;113(5):545–554. https://doi.org/10.2105/AJPH.2023.307230)

AJPH May 2023, Vol 113, No. 5

The REal-time Assessment of Community Transmission-1 (REACT-1) Study sought to provide reliable and timely estimates of severe acute respiratory syndrome coronavirus 2 (SARS-CoV-2) infection prevalence and data on associated symptoms and covariates from random samples of the population of England.

DATA SYSTEM

This study involved 19 distinct rounds of data collection, from May 1, 2020, to March 31, 2022 (Figure 1).

Name and Sponsor of the Program

The REACT-1 Study is funded by the Department of Health and Social Care in England.

Purpose

The aim of REACT-1 was to rapidly detect changes in SARS-CoV-2 transmission in England and to give early warning of any upturn in infections. As well as providing reliable estimates of prevalence of SARS-CoV-2 infection over time, by person and place, REACT-1 gave estimates of vaccine effectiveness against infection and identified new variants as they emerged in the population.

Public Health Significance

When REACT-1 was established during the first lockdown in England, little was known about the spread of SARS-CoV-2 in the population, who was most at risk, when infection rates were rising or

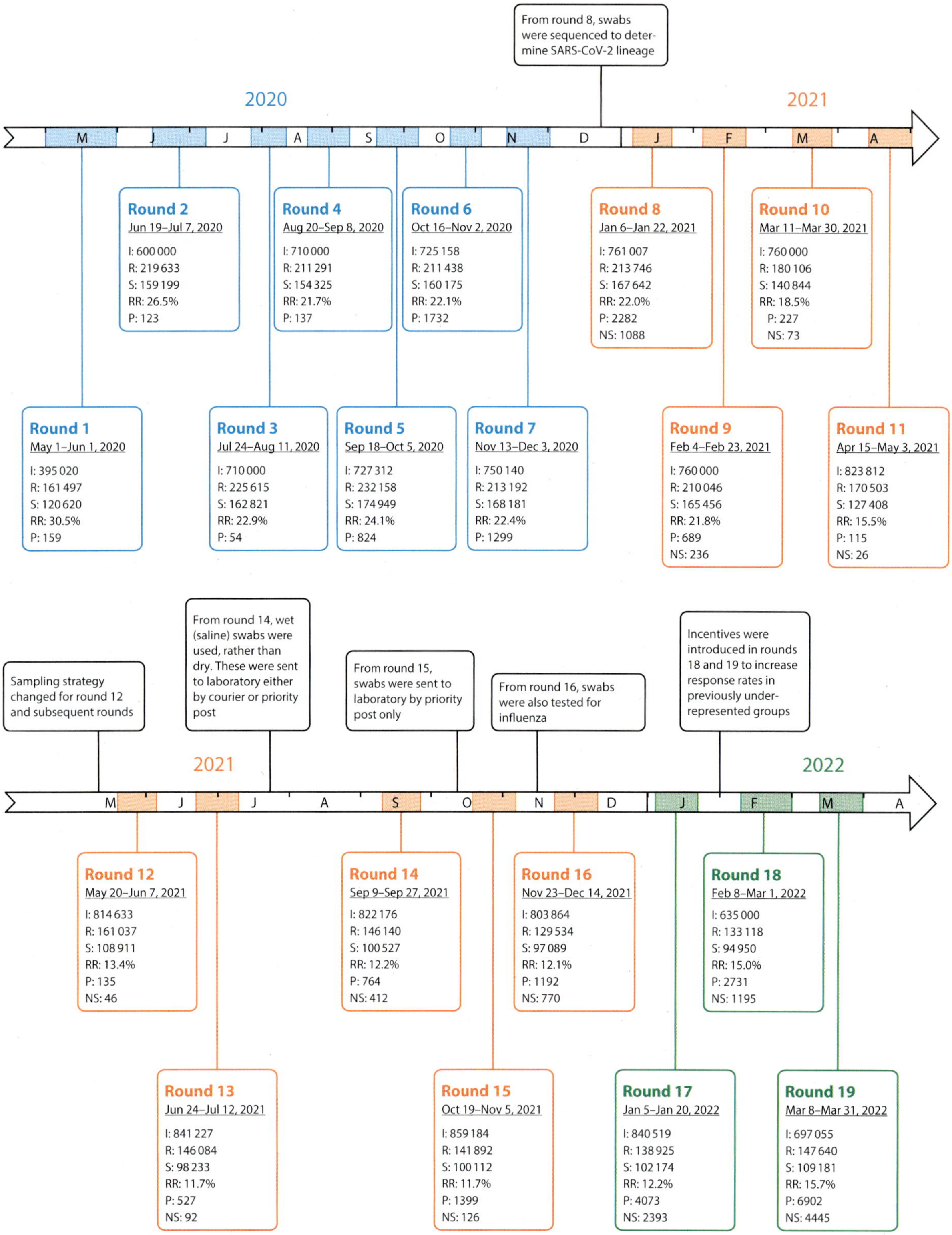

FIGURE 1— REACT-1 Study Timeline Over 19 Rounds of Data Collection: England, May 1, 2020–March 31, 2022

Note. REACT-1 = REal-time Assessment of Community Transmission-1; SARS-CoV-2 = severe acute respiratory syndrome coronavirus 2. For each round, we report the number of invitations sent (I), the number of participants registered (R), the number of valid swabs received (S), and response rate (RR), as defined by the number of valid swabs over the number of invitations sent and the total number of SARS-CoV-2–positive swabs (P) these yielded. From round 8 onward (from January 6, 2021), viral sequencing was also available, and we report the number of SARS-CoV-2 (sub)-lineages determined per round (NS).

falling, and where—for example, at national, regional, or subregional levels. REACT-1 was designed to provide rapid information on the time course of the infection, geographic spread (at high spatial resolution), and estimates of the reproduction number R.[1,2] These data were given directly to the government as they were obtained to inform the public health response and enable timely implementation of public health interventions.

DATA COLLECTION/ PROCESSING

The study tested self-obtained throat and nose swabs from random samples of the population of England for presence of SARS-CoV-2, using reverse-transcriptase polymerase chain reaction (rt-PCR). Participants also completed a self-administered questionnaire, either online or by telephone. In later rounds, we carried out viral genome sequencing to obtain information on circulating variants.

Data Sources and Collection Mode

Source population. The study team (researchers from Imperial College London and its logistics partner Ipsos) invited random cross-sectional samples of individuals aged 5 years and older in England by mail to participate in REACT-1.

Registration. We invited named individuals on the National Health Service (NHS) list of patients to register for the study either online or by telephone. For participants, we obtained from the NHS register their name, sex, general practitioner practice code, address and residential postcode, mobile (cell) telephone number, e-mail address (for early rounds only), date of birth (to round 7, November 13 to December 3, 2020) or month and year of birth (subsequent rounds), and NHS number.

Questionnaires. Participants completed a brief questionnaire at registration either online or by telephone and a further, more detailed questionnaire for those who provided a swab. These included information on household composition; key worker status; social behaviors (e.g., mask wearing, commuting); contact with a person known or suspected to have COVID-19; whether, at time of survey, participants had experienced 1 or more of a list of symptoms and timing of the symptoms (participants not reporting symptoms may have developed symptoms later, but these were not captured); symptoms lasting more than 4 weeks; self-reported long COVID; and self-reported height and weight, smoking, vaccination history, and attitudes toward vaccination. Participants were asked for consent for recontact and for longer-term follow-up through linkage to their NHS records including data from the national immunization program. The questionnaires are available on the study Web site.[3]

Swabs. Individuals who registered for the study received a swab kit by mail, with both written and video instructions provided for collecting a self-obtained throat and nose swab (by parent or guardian for children aged 5–12 years). During the first round of data collection (May 1 to June 1, 2020), swabs were initially collected in viral transport medium and sent to 1 of 4 Public Health England laboratories for processing (n = 8595 swabs with reported result). All subsequent collections during round 1 to round 13 (June 24 to July 12, 2021) were obtained by using dry swabs. Participants were asked to obtain and refrigerate the sample and request a courier pick-up (same or next day) for sample collection. To maintain sample integrity, samples were then transported to a central hub before daily shipping to a commercial laboratory, all within a cold chain (4° to 8°C) for testing for presence of SARS-CoV-2.

For round 14 (September 9–27, 2021), we modified the way swab samples were handled, switching to wet swabs in saline solution. We randomized on a 1-to-1 basis whether samples were sent to the laboratory by priority mail or were picked up by courier without the cold chain (although samples were refrigerated on arrival at the depot before onward transportation to the laboratory). There was a slightly higher return rate for samples handled by mail, although prevalence estimates were slightly higher and cycle threshold (Ct) values among positives slightly lower (indicating slightly better preservation) in the samples sent by courier compared with samples shipped by mail.[4] In subsequent rounds from round 15 (October 19 to November 5, 2021), we switched to shipment by priority mail in saline solution only for all swabs.

Ethical Procedures

Ethics. We obtained ethics approval from the South Central–Berkshire B Research Ethics Committee (IRAS ID: 283787). Participants gave individual consent to take part, either online or by telephone (parent or guardian for children aged 5–12 years and for those aged 13–17 years where parent or guardian completed registration on behalf of the child).

Public involvement. A public advisory panel provides input into the design, conduct, and dissemination of the REACT research program. We have a data access committee with lay representation.

Population and Geographic Coverage

Population coverage. The target population was the population of England aged 5 years and older. We designed the study to provide robust estimates of prevalence at regional and subregional level, including estimates at lower-tier local authority (LTLA) level. We included data for 316 of the 317 LTLAs in England excluding the Isles of Scilly (after the first round), and by combining data for the City of London with Westminster, we report results across 315 LTLAs overall. At each round, we provided national and regional estimates of epidemic growth, and prevalence estimates for key demographic subgroups including by age, ethnicity, household size, occupation, and socioeconomic status. Smoothed estimates of weighted prevalence over the 19 rounds of the study (May 1, 2020, to March 31, 2022) by age and region, as well as overall, are shown in Figure 2.

Sampling frame. We used the list of patients aged 5 years and older registered in the NHS with a general practitioner in England (near-universal population coverage). We obtained a new random sample at each round from data on the NHS register held centrally by NHS Digital.

Sampling strategy. For rounds 1 to 11 (between May 1, 2020, and May 3, 2021), we aimed to obtain LTLA-stratified random samples with approximately equal numbers of participants in each of the 315 LTLAs to enable local estimates of prevalence across England. From round 12 onward, we adjusted the sampling procedure to select the sample randomly in proportion to population at the LTLA level, because urban and inner-city areas (which tended to have higher infection rates) were relatively underrepresented in comparison with more sparsely populated rural areas.

Unit of Data Collection and Sample Size

Unit of data collection. Data collection was at the individual level. Named, randomly selected individuals were invited to take part; the invitation was nontransferable to other members of the family or household.

Sample size and response rates. Over the 19 rounds of the study, a total of 2 512 797 valid swabs were included from among 14 036 117 invitations, giving an overall response rate (number of valid swabs/number of invitations sent out) of 17.9%. Sample size by round varied from 94 950 in round 18 (February 8 to March 1, 2022, when prevalence rates were very high; Figure 2) to 168 181 in round 7 (November 13 to December 3, 2020). Response rates also varied by round, ranging from 11.7% in rounds 13 (June 24 to July 12, 2021) and 15 (October 19 to November 5, 2021) to 30.5% in round 1 (May 1 to June 1, 2020, during the first lockdown in England).

To maximize response rates, with our logistics partner Ipsos, we implemented a series of reminders to improve both registration rates and swab and survey return rates among those registering to take part. For registration, we included up to 4 reminders by letter, text, or (in 2 rounds) mobile phone contact. Among people who had requested a swab kit but not returned the swab or symptom survey, from round 3 (July 24 to August 11, 2020) Ipsos used a series of up to 3 reminders by either e-mail or text (or letter where an e-mail address or mobile phone number were not provided). A reminder by phone call was added from round 12 onward (May 20 to June 7, 2021) where a mobile phone number was provided at registration. Overall, a substantial proportion of those registering and those returning a swab did so following one of these reminders.

In addition, following a successful pilot in which different incentives (£10 to £30) were offered (in a randomized evaluation) to a subsample of people taking part in round 15, we added an incentive in rounds 18 (February 8 to March 1, 2022) and 19 (March 8–31, 2022) to increase response rates among underrepresented groups. For returning their completed test, those aged 13 to 17 and 35 to 44 years were offered a gift voucher worth £10 while those aged 18 to 34 years were offered a voucher worth £20. This had the effect of increasing the response rate in these groups, with the overall response rate in rounds 18 and 19 rising to 15.0% and 15.7%, respectively (Figure 1).

Completeness. We obtained sufficient data by round to be able to estimate prevalence by age, sex, region, and other key demographic groups including ethnicity, occupation, household size, and socioeconomic status (as determined by an area-level deprivation score).

Generalizability. We weighted the data at each round (see subsequent "Prevalence estimates and random iterative method weighting" section) to be representative of England as a whole and to provide unbiased estimates of prevalence that were comparable across rounds, including with the change in sampling strategy to be in proportion to population size. The ratio of weighted to unweighted prevalence gives an indication as to the potential

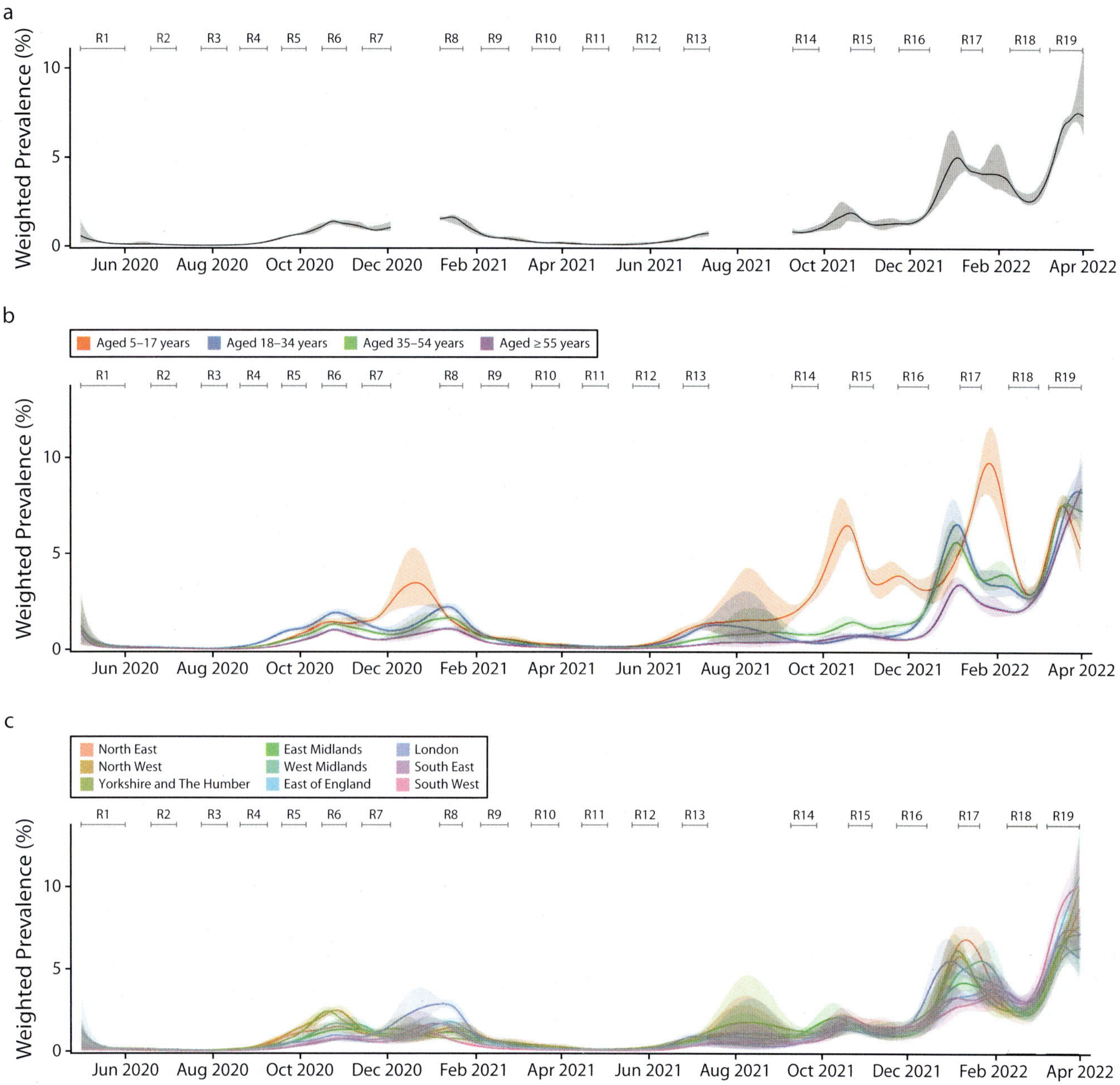

FIGURE 2— Smoothed Weighted SARS-CoV-2 Swab-Positivity Prevalence From All Rounds of the REACT-1 Study by (a) Overall Prevalence, (b) Age Groups, and (c) Region: England, May 1, 2020–March 31, 2022

Note. REACT-1 = REal-time Assessment of Community Transmission-1; SARS-CoV-2 = severe acute respiratory syndrome coronavirus 2. We used the random iterative method (RIM) weighting approach to correct for possible nonresponse bias and ensure that our prevalence estimates were representative of the population of England as a whole. Using a Bayesian penalized-spline model fit to the daily swab-positivity data, we estimated the median (plain line) and 95% credible intervals (shaded regions) of weighted prevalence throughout the study period. Results are shown for the full population of England (A) with model fit on rounds 1–7, 8–13, and 14–19, separately, and for 4 broad age groups (B): 5–17 y, 18–34 y, 35–54 y, and 55 y and older, and by region (C), with model fit throughout the duration of the study. Ranking of weighted prevalence by age and region changed over the course of the epidemic in England. For example, there was particularly high prevalence in those aged 5 to 17 y in October 2021 and January 2022.

bias introduced by nonresponse in different demographic groups. This ratio was consistently above 1 for rounds 1 to 17 (i.e., unweighted prevalence was consistently below the expected rates for England). However, the variability around the ratio tended to decrease following the change in sampling strategy implemented in round 12, and the ratio itself fell to 1 (i.e., no bias on average) in both rounds 18 and 19, reflecting the use of incentives in those

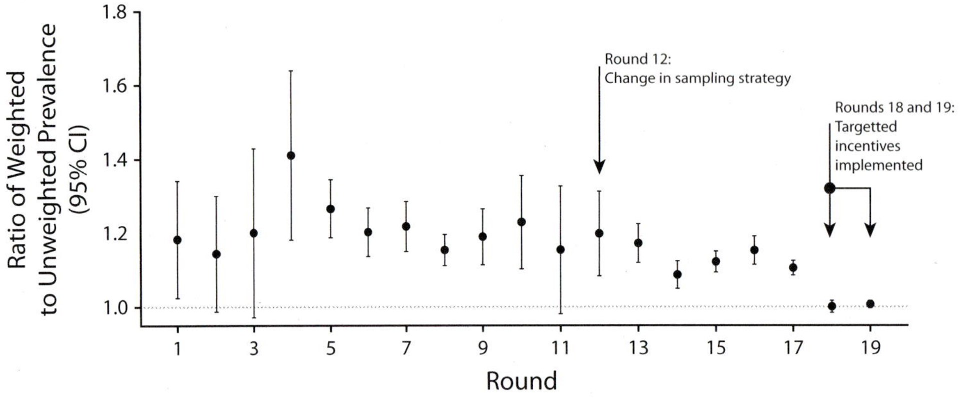

FIGURE 3— **Per-Round Ratio of Weighted Over Unweighted Prevalence of SARS-CoV-2 Swab Positivity in REACT-1 Over 19 Rounds: England, May 1, 2020–March 31, 2022**

Note. SARS-CoV-2 = severe acute respiratory syndrome coronavirus 2. We report the mean and 95% confidence intervals (CIs) for the ratio.

rounds among harder-to-reach younger people (Figure 3).

Surveillance Design and Data Collection Frequency

We designed the study to recruit a series of representative cross-sectional samples of the population of England aged 5 years and older. As noted, we carried out data collection over a 23-month period from May 1, 2020, to March 31, 2022, through a series of distinct rounds that took place over a 2- to 3-week period approximately monthly—exceptions were gaps between rounds 7 and 8 over Christmas 2020 and between rounds 13 and 14 during summer 2021 (Figure 2). The data were collected prospectively and reported in near-real-time. Where possible, we aimed to obtain independent samples at each round (i.e., sampling without replacement); however, given the scale of the sampling efforts (around one quarter of the population of England was invited) this could not always be achieved, and around 3% of the study population took part more than once.

Key Data Elements and Data Quality/Editing

Prevalence estimates and random iterative method weighting. We used random iterative method (RIM) weighting[5] to correct for bias in (unweighted) prevalence estimates introduced by varying nonresponse in different demographic groups, taking account of age–sex categories, deciles of an area-level index of multiple deprivation,[6] LTLA population counts, and ethnicity. We obtained age, sex, and LTLA counts from the Office for National Statistics midyear population estimates,[7] counts by ethnic group from the Labour Force Survey,[8] and index of multiple deprivation deciles from linkage to residential postcodes using the NHS digital sampling frame. We based the RIM weighting on proportions rather than population totals, with age grouped into 9 categories: 5–12; 13–17; 18–24; 25–34; 35–44; 45–54; 55–64; 65–74; and 75 years or older, giving 18 age–sex categories. Self-reported ethnicity was grouped into 9 categories: White, mixed/multiple ethnic groups, Indian, Pakistani, Bangladeshi, Chinese, any other Asian background, Black African/Caribbean/other, and any other ethnic group or missing.

For the RIM weighting (first stage) we weighted each sample to LTLA counts and age–sex categories only, with adjustment to ensure that the final weighted estimates were as close as possible to the source population. Then, using the first stage weights as starting weights, we adjusted the RIM weighting for all 4 weighting variables, trimming the adjustment factor between the first and second stage weights at the first and 99th percentiles to dampen the extreme weights. We calculated the final weights as the first stage weights multiplied by the trimmed adjustment factor for the second stage, with credible intervals for weighted prevalence estimates calculated using the "survey" package in R.[9]

Time trends and smoothed prevalence. To analyze time trends in swab positivity, we used an exponential model of growth or decay assuming that the daily weighted number of positive samples (out of the daily weighted total number of samples) arose from a binomial distribution. The model is of the form $I(t) = I_0.e^{rt}$, where $I(t)$ is the swab positivity at time t, I_0 is swab positivity at the

AJPH May 2023, Vol 113, No. 5

beginning of data collection per round, and r is the growth rate. On a given day, the binomial likelihood for P (out of N) positive tests is then $P \sim B(N, I_0.e^{rt})$ based on day of swabbing or, if unavailable, day of sample collection. We used a bivariate No-U-Turn sampler to estimate posterior credible intervals assuming uniform prior distributions on I_0 and r.[10]

To fit a smoothed trend (Figure 2), we used a Bayesian penalized-spline model[11] to the daily data using a No-U-Turn Sampler in logit space, splitting the data into segments of approximately 5 days by regularly spaced knots, with further knots included beyond the period of the study to remove edge effects. We defined a system of 4th-order basis-splines (b-splines) over the knots, with a model comprising a linear combination of these b-splines. We guarded against overfitting through inclusion of a second-order random-walk prior distribution on the coefficients of the b-splines. This prior distribution takes the form $b_i = 2b_{i-1} - b_{i-2} + u_i$, where b_i is the ith b-spline coefficient and u_i is normally distributed with $u_i \sim N(0,\rho^2)$. The prior distribution assumes a constant first derivative and therefore penalizes against changes in growth rate unless supported by the data. The penalization of changes in growth rate is controlled by the parameter ρ, assigned an inverse γ prior distribution, $\rho \sim IG(0.001, 0.001)$. We assumed a uniform prior distribution on the first 2 b-spline coefficients.

Laboratory procedures. Swabs were sent by courier (earlier rounds) or by priority mail (later rounds) to a depot for onward transport to a single commercial laboratory for analysis by rt-PCR. The laboratory analyzed extracted nucleic acid for SARS-CoV-2 with the ViroBOAR 1·0 RT-qPCR kit (EuroFins Genomics, GmbH, Ebersberg, Germany) and on the Roche Lightcycler 480 II (Roche Diagnostics, Almere, The Netherlands) to detect in parallel 2 gene targets: N gene and E gene. The assay has a specificity close to 100% with limit of detection of 10 copies per microliter. In addition, the laboratory developed a multiplex for influenza A and B, which was added in November 2021 (Figure 1). Performance of the multiplex was tested against an established assay (Luminex NxTAG Respiratory Pathogen Panel, Luminex Corporation, Austin, Texas, USA) in an independent commercial laboratory, as well against sequencing of selected samples in the UK Health Security Agency laboratories.

Cycle threshold and laboratory calibration experiments. We used Ct values as a proxy for viral load for the 2 SARS-CoV-2 gene targets (N gene and E gene). The rt-PCR was considered positive if both gene targets were detected or if N gene was detected with Ct value less than 37. This Ct threshold was determined following 3 separate calibration experiments. In the first, we sent RNA extraction plates (n = 10) from the commercial laboratory to 2 UK Accreditation Service–accredited laboratories for blinded reanalysis. We found concordant results for 919 negative samples and all 40 controls. We detected viral RNA in 11 of the 19 samples with a Ct value reported positive by the commercial laboratory (N gene Ct value ranging from 16.5 to 40.7); in 10 of these 11 samples, N gene Ct value was less than 37.

Second, in a serial dilution experiment of synthetic SARS-CoV-2 RNA, the commercial laboratory detected 2.5 copies at Ct 38; also, while following serial dilution of known positive samples with low viral load, the commercial laboratory identified an N gene signal at Ct greater than 37 in most instances.

Third, a Public Health England reference laboratory reanalyzed a further 40 unblinded positive samples with N gene Ct values greater than 35 (range = 35.7–46.8) and without a signal for E gene, detecting SARS-CoV-2 RNA in 15 of 40 (38%) samples (2 of 4 with N gene Ct value < 37). We then consolidated the results of all 3 calibration experiments to set the positivity criteria noted previously, which we used throughout each round of REACT-1.

Viral genome sequencing. We undertook viral genome sequencing to provide information on specific variants from round 8 (January 6–22, 2021) onward. The Quadram Institute, in Norwich, UK, carried out the sequencing for samples that tested positive on rt-PCR with Ct value of (variously) 34 or below, or 32 or below, in either the N or E gene, and with sufficient volume of sample available. The Quadram Institute used the ARTIC protocol[12] for viral RNA amplification, CoronaHiT for preparation of sequencing libraries,[13] and the ARTIC bioinformatics pipeline,[14] and assigned lineages by using PangoLEARN.[15] Transitions of each of the variants during the course of the epidemic in the United Kingdom and their detection in England in the REACT-1 study are shown in Figure 4.

Managing disclosure risks. To protect confidentiality, individual data are not released, and tabular data are suppressed if there are fewer than 5 entries in a cell where 1 or more is a positive for SARS-CoV-2.

DATA ANALYSIS/ DISSEMINATION

The data collected in REACT-1 were analyzed and reported in real-time to

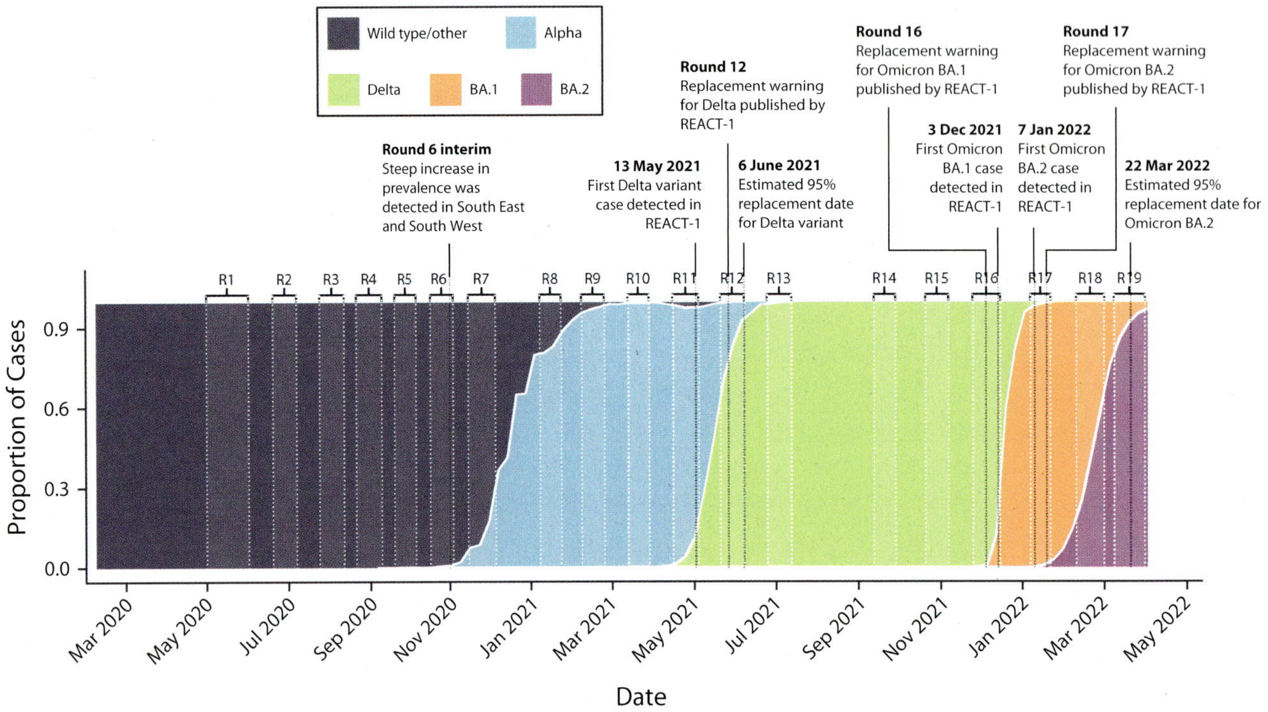

FIGURE 4— Proportion of Wild Type, Alpha, and Delta Lineages and Omicron BA.1 and Omicron BA.2 Sublineages: GISAID, United Kingdom, April 1, 2022

Note. GISAID = Global Initiative on Sharing Avian Influenza Data; R = round; REACT-1 = REal-time Assessment of Community Transmission-1. For Delta lineage and Omicron BA.1 and Omicron BA.2 sublineages, we report the date of first detection in REACT-1 samples with determined lineage, the date at which REACT-1 reported a possible variant replacement, and the corresponding estimated date of replacement as defined by the date at which the estimated median proportion of the given variant was greater than 95%.

government and widely disseminated in timely fashion to the scientific community and the public.

Interpretation Issues

Over the course of the study, we observed a gradual decline in response rates, from a high of 30.5% in round 1 (May 1 to June 1, 2020), carried out during the first lockdown in England when it was very difficult to get a diagnostic test through other means. We were able to offset some of the decline in response by including a modest monetary incentive (via gift voucher) to people aged 13 to 44 years who are harder to reach in surveys. Moreover, our reported response rates are conservative estimates as we based them on numbers of swabs with a valid rt-PCR result compared with the numbers of invitation letters sent out, some of which may not have reached (or been opened by) the recipient. We used RIM weighting to correct the sample to be representative of the population of England as a whole. Nonetheless, to the extent that this relied on weighting factors, some bias may have been introduced into our estimates of prevalence, particularly when examining effects in specific groups (e.g., by occupation, ethnicity, or deprivation).

Changes in the way the swab samples were collected, transported, and tested may have introduced small differences across rounds, although these should not have affected within-round trends in prevalence. The switch from dry to wet (saline) swabs and from collection of samples with to without a cold chain might have affected diagnostic sensitivity. Because of financial and logistical constraints, we were not able to directly compare dry swab transported by courier on a cold chain, as was used before round 14, with wet swab sent by priority mail, which was used from round 15 on (Figure 1). However, we were reassured by the small differences between the samples collected by mail and courier in our randomized comparison during round 14.

More than 2 million people consented to data linkage to their NHS records, but for the remainder, we are unable to obtain hospitalizations or mortality data, or accurate vaccination data from the national COVID-19 immunization program. Although we do have self-report data on vaccination history, for those without linked data, dates of vaccination and vaccine type may be missing or less reliable than in the linked data, which may introduce bias. Furthermore, those who do and do not consent to data linkage might differ in important ways, such as social mixing patterns.

Linkage Ability

Participants were asked whether they consented to linkage to their health records. For participants with consent, data linkage (based on their unique NHS number) includes vaccine history (vaccine type and date) and outcome data (hospitalizations, deaths).

Data Release/Accessibility

Access to REACT-1 individual-level data are restricted to protect participants' anonymity. Summary statistics, descriptive tables, and code from REACT-1 are available at https://github.com/mrc-ide/reactidd. REACT-1 study materials are available for each round at https://www.imperial.ac.uk/medicine/research-and-impact/groups/react-study/for-researchers/react-1-study-materials.

Key References/Other Information

We have published our protocol[16] and on our findings during the 23 months of fieldwork, including methodological work on estimation of growth rates and reproduction number, on transitions between variants, and on the duration of swab-positivity after infection.[1,2,4,17–25] We also published preprints giving results for each round. Links to all our publications are given on our Web site at https://www.imperial.ac.uk/medicine/research-and-impact/groups/react-study/real-time-assessment-of-community-transmission-findings.

PUBLIC HEALTH IMPLICATIONS

REACT-1 provided reliable and robust estimates of the prevalence of SARS-CoV-2 infection and of epidemic growth of COVID-19 in England. We provided prevalence estimates (and odds ratios) for different sociodemographic groups—for example, by age, sex, ethnicity, occupation, household size, and deprivation—and estimates of vaccine effectiveness against infection. The government used these data to inform the public health response across nearly 2 years of the epidemic in England.

Impact

Unlike the routine testing data, results from REACT-1 were not dependent on the availability of tests, which affected prevalence estimates in the routine surveillance data,[22] nor were they biased by test-seeking behaviors, and importantly included asymptomatic as well as symptomatic infections, which is critical in understanding the infection dynamics.[26] The results of REACT-1 were reported at least weekly to the government to provide situational awareness and inform policy and public health interventions. Thus, REACT-1 informed the timing of the second national lockdown in England, reinforced the need for the "rule of 6" (i.e., no more than 6 people allowed at social gatherings), provided key data underpinning school closure policy, and contributed to recommendations to protect those living in large households. REACT-1 was one of the first studies to detect the rapid rise of infections in southeast London, Kent, and Essex in September 2021[27] as the Alpha variant began to take hold and reported the rapid replacement of the Alpha variant by Delta in May 2021,[24] Delta by Omicron BA.1 in December 2021,[20] and Omicron BA.1 by Omicron BA.2 in February to March 2022[19] (Figure 4).

In addition to our role in providing situational awareness to government, we placed REACT-1 data into the public domain in near-real-time (through both preprints and press releases and the media), thus informing both the international scientific community and the public as to the current state of the epidemic in England. AJPH

ABOUT THE AUTHORS

Paul Elliott, Matthew Whitaker, David Tang, Oliver Eales, Barbara Bodinier, Haowei Wang, Christina Atchison, Deborah Ashby, Helen Ward, and Marc Chadeu-Hyam are with the School of Public Health, Imperial College London, UK. Nicholas Steyn and Christl A. Donnelly are with the Department of Statistics, University of Oxford, Oxford, UK. Joshua Elliott is with the Imperial College Healthcare NHS Trust, London. Ara Darzi is with the Institute of Global Health Innovation, Imperial College London. Wendy Barclay, Graham Taylor, and Graham S. Cooke are with the Department of Infectious Disease, Imperial College London.

CORRESPONDENCE

Correspondence should be sent to Professor Paul Elliott, School of Public Health, Imperial College London, St Mary's campus, London W2 1PG, UK (e-mail: p.elliott@imperial.ac.uk). Reprints can be ordered at https://ajph.org by clicking the "Reprints" link.

PUBLICATION INFORMATION

Full Citation: Elliott P, Whitaker M, Tang D, et al. Design and implementation of a national SARS-CoV-2 monitoring program in England: REACT-1 study. *Am J Public Health*. 2023;113(5):545–554.

Acceptance Date: January 10, 2023.

DOI: https://doi.org/10.2105/AJPH.2023.307230

CONTRIBUTORS

P. Elliott drafted the article. The other authors critically reviewed the article and provided comments. All authors agreed to submission for publication.

ACKNOWLEDGMENTS

This study was funded by the Department of Health and Social Care in England. P. Elliott is director of the MRC Centre for Environment and Health (MR/L01341X/1 and MR/S019669/1). P. Elliott acknowledges support from Health Data Research UK; the National Institute for Health and Care Research (NIHR) Imperial Biomedical Research Centre; NIHR Health Protection Research Units in Chemical and Radiation Threats and Hazards, and Environmental Exposures and Health; the British Heart Foundation Centre for Research Excellence at Imperial College London (RE/18/4/34215); and the UK Dementia Research Institute at Imperial College London (MC_PC_17114). N. Steyn acknowledges support from the Oxford-Radcliffe Scholarship from University College, Oxford, and the Engineering and Physical Sciences Research Council Centre for Doctoral Training in Modern Statistics and Statistical Machine Learning (Imperial College London and University of Oxford). We thank A. Maslov for supporting this research through studentship support for N. Steyn. H. Ward acknowledges support from an NIHR Senior Investigator Award, the Wellcome Trust (205456/Z/16/Z), and the NIHR Applied Research Collaboration North West London. J. Elliott is an NIHR academic clinical fellow in infectious diseases. G. S. Cooke is supported by an NIHR professorship. C. A. Donnelly acknowledges support from the MRC Centre for Global Infectious Disease Analysis, the NIHR Health Protection Research Unit in Emerging and Zoonotic Infections, and the NIHR-funded Vaccine Efficacy Evaluation for Priority Emerging Diseases (PR-OD-1017-20007). M. Chadeau-Hyam and B. Bodinier acknowledge support from Cancer Research UK, Population Research Committee Project grant "Mechanomics" (grant 22184 to M. Chadeu-Hyam). M. Chadeu-Hyam acknowledges support from the H2020-EXPANSE (Horizon 2020 grant 874627) and H2020-LongITools (Horizon 2020 grant 874739).

We thank key collaborators on this work: K. Beaver, S. Clemens, G. Welch, N. Gilby, K. Ward, G. Pantelidou, and K. Pickering at Ipsos; G. Fontana and J. Alford at the Institute of Global Health Innovation at Imperial College London; E. Johnson, R. Elliott, and G. Blakoe at the School of Public Health, Imperial College London; and A. J. Page and N.-F. Alikhan at the Quadram Institute, Norwich, UK. We also thank North West London Pathology and Public Health England (now UK Health Security Agency) for help in calibration of the laboratory analyses, Patient Experience Research Centre at Imperial College London and the REACT Public Advisory Panel, NHS Digital for access to the NHS register, and the Department of Health and Social Care for logistical support.

Note. The funders had no role in the design and conduct of the study; collection, management, analysis, and interpretation of the data; and preparation, review, or approval of this article.

CONFLICTS OF INTEREST

MC-H holds shares in the O-SMOSE company. Consulting activities conducted by the company are independent of the present work, and MC-H has no conflicts of interest to declare. All other authors have no competing interests to declare.

HUMAN PARTICIPANT PROTECTION

The REACT-1 study received ethical approval from the South Central–Berkshire B Research Ethics Committee, UK.

REFERENCES

1. Eales O, Ainslie KEC, Walters CE, et al. Appropriately smoothing prevalence data to inform estimates of growth rate and reproduction number. *Epidemics.* 2022;40:100604. https://doi.org/10.1016/j.epidem.2022.100604
2. Eales O, Walters CE, Wang H, et al. Characterising the persistence of RT-PCR positivity and incidence in a community survey of SARS-CoV-2. *Wellcome Open Res.* 2022;7:102. https://doi.org/10.12688/wellcomeopenres.17723.1
3. REACT 1 study materials. Imperial College London. Available at: https://www.imperial.ac.uk/medicine/research-and-impact/groups/react-study/for-researchers/react-1-study-materials. Accessed January 1, 2023.
4. Chadeau-Hyam M, Wang H, Eales O, et al. SARS-CoV-2 infection and vaccine effectiveness in England (REACT-1): a series of cross-sectional random community surveys. *Lancet Respir Med.* 2022;10(4):355–366. https://doi.org/10.1016/S2213-2600(21)00542-7
5. Sharot T. Weighting survey results. Available at: http://www.redresearch.com/wp/wp-content/uploads/2016/01/Weighting-Survey-Results.pdf. Accessed April 5, 2022.
6. McLennan D, Noble S, Noble M, Plunkett E, Wright, GN. *The English Indices of Deprivation 2019.* Ministry of Housing, Communities, and Local Government September 2019. Available at: https://assets.publishing.service.gov.uk/government/uploads/system/uploads/attachment_data/file/833951/IoD2019_Technical_Report.pdf. Accessed January 1, 2023.
7. Population estimates for the UK, England and Wales, Scotland and Northern Ireland: mid-2020. Newport, Wales: Office for National Statistics; June 25, 2021.
8. Labour Force Survey. Office for National Statistics. Available at: https://www.ons.gov.uk/surveys/informationforhouseholdsandindividuals/householdandindividualsurveys/labourforcesurvey. Accessed January 1, 2023.
9. Lumley T. Analysis of complex survey samples. *J Stat Softw.* 2004;9(8):1–19. https://doi.org/10.18637/jss.v009.i08
10. Hoffman MD, Gelman A. The No-U-Turn sampler: adaptively setting path lengths in Hamiltonian Monte Carlo. *J Mach Learn Res.* 2014;15:1593–1623. Available at: https://www.jmlr.org/papers/volume15/hoffman14a/hoffman14a.pdf. Accessed January 1, 2023.
11. Lang S, Brezger A. Bayesian P-Splines. *J Comput Graph Stat.* 2004;13(1):183–212. https://doi.org/10.1198/1061860043010
12. Quick J. nCoV-2019 sequencing protocol v3 (LoCost). Available at: https://www.protocols.io/view/ncov-2019-sequencing-protocol-v3-locost-bp2l6n26rgqe/v3. Accessed January 1, 2023.
13. Baker DJ, Aydin A, Le-Viet T, et al. CoronaHiT: high-throughput sequencing of SARS-CoV-2 genomes. *Genome Med.* 2021;13(1):21. https://doi.org/10.1186/s13073-021-00839-5
14. A Nextflow Pipeline for Running the ARTIC Network's Field Bioinformatics Tools. GitHub. Available at: https://github.com/connor-lab. Accessed January 1, 2023.
15. Pangolin: Software Package for Assigning SARS-CoV-2 Genome Sequences to Global Lineages. Github. Available at: https://github.com/cov-lineages/pangolin. Accessed January 20, 2022.
16. Riley S, Atchison C, Ashby D, et al. REal-time Assessment of Community Transmission (REACT) of SARS-CoV-2 virus: study protocol. *Wellcome Open Res.* 2021;5:200. https://doi.org/10.12688/wellcomeopenres.16228.2
17. Elliott P, Eales O, Bodinier B, et al. Dynamics of a national Omicron SARS-CoV-2 epidemic during January 2022 in England. *Nat Commun.* 2022;13(1):4500. https://doi.org/10.1038/s41467-022-32121-6
18. Eales O, de Oliveira Martins L, Page AJ, et al. Dynamics of competing SARS-CoV-2 variants during the Omicron epidemic in England. *Nat Commun.* 2022;13(1):4375. https://doi.org/10.1038/s41467-022-32096-4
19. Elliott P, Eales O, Steyn N, et al. Twin peaks: the Omicron SARS-CoV-2 BA.1 and BA.2 epidemics in England. *Science.* 2022;376(6600):eabq4411. https://doi.org/10.1126/science.abq4411
20. Elliott P, Bodinier B, Eales O, et al. Rapid increase in Omicron infections in England during December 2021: REACT-1 study. *Science.* 2022;375(6587):1406–1411. https://doi.org/10.1126/science.abn8347
21. Chadeau-Hyam M, Tang D, Eales O, et al. Omicron SARS-CoV-2 epidemic in England during February 2022: a series of cross-sectional community surveys. *Lancet Reg Health Eur.* 2022;21:100462. https://doi.org/10.1016/j.lanepe.2022.100462
22. Riley S, Ainslie KEC, Eales O, et al. Resurgence of SARS-CoV-2: detection by community viral surveillance. *Science.* 2021;372(6545):990–995. https://doi.org/10.1126/science.abf0874
23. Chadeau-Hyam M, Eales O, Bodinier B, et al. Breakthrough SARS-CoV-2 infections in double and triple vaccinated adults and single dose vaccine effectiveness among children in autumn 2021 in England: REACT-1 study. *EClinicalMedicine.* 2022;48:101419. https://doi.org/10.1016/j.eclinm.2022.101419
24. Elliott P, Haw D, Wang H, et al. Exponential growth, high prevalence of SARS-CoV-2, and vaccine effectiveness associated with the Delta variant. *Science.* 2021;374(6574):eabl9551. https://doi.org/10.1126/science.abl9551
25. Eales O, Wang H, Haw D, et al. Trends in SARS-CoV-2 infection prevalence during England's roadmap out of lockdown, January to July 2021. *PLOS Comput Biol.* 2022;18(11):e1010724. https://doi.org/10.1371/journal.pcbi.1010724
26. Oran DP, Topol EJ. The proportion of SARS-CoV-2 infections that are asymptomatic. *Ann Intern Med.* 2021;174(9):1344–1345. https://doi.org/10.7326/L21-0491
27. Riley S, Ainslie KEC, Eales O, et al. High prevalence of SARS-CoV-2 swab positivity and increasing R number in England during October 2020: REACT-1 round 6 interim report. *medRxiv.* Published online November 3, 2020. https://doi.org/10.1101/2020.10.30.20223123

Wildfire Threat to Inpatient Health Care Facilities in California, 2022

Neil Singh Bedi, BA, Caleb Dresser, MD, MPH, Akash Yadav, MSc, Andrew Schroeder, PhD, MPP, and Satchit Balsari, MD, MPH

Objectives. To assess wildfire risks to California inpatient health care facilities in 2022.

Methods. Locations of inpatient facilities and associated inpatient bed capacities were mapped in relation to California Department of Forestry and Fire Protection fire threat zones (FTZs), which combine expected fire frequency with potential fire behavior. We computed the distances of each facility to the nearest high, very high, and extreme FTZs.

Results. Half (107 290 beds) of California's total inpatient capacity is within 0.87 miles of a high FTZ and 95% (203 665 beds) is within 3.7 miles of a high FTZ. Half of the total inpatient capacity is within 3.3 miles of a very high FTZ and 15.5 miles of an extreme FTZ.

Conclusions. Wildfires threaten a large number of inpatient health care facilities in California. In many counties, all health care facilities may be at risk.

Public Health Implications. Wildfires in California are rapid-onset disasters with short preimpact phases. Policies should address facility-level preparedness including smoke mitigation, sheltering measures, evacuation procedures, and resource allocation. Regional evacuation needs, including access to emergency medical services and patient transportation, must also be considered. (*Am J Public Health.* 2023;113(5):555–558. https://doi.org/10.2105/AJPH.2023.307236)

AJPH May 2023, Vol 113, No. 5

California is experiencing an intensifying wildfire crisis. Of the 20 largest wildfires in the state's history, all but 3 took place in the past 2 decades, with 7 occurring in 2020 and 2021.[1] Wildfires pose a threat to the structural integrity, operations, and accessibility of health care facilities, accounting for 18.4% of hospital evacuations in the United States during the 21st century.[2] Recent examples in California include evacuations from hospitals in Sonoma County, sometimes twice within the same fire season.[3] Inpatient facility evacuations are a complex process and often require coordination across health systems and jurisdictions. They can pose a danger to patients and staff, even when advance warning is available.[4,5] In this article, we use publicly available data to assess the burden of wildfire risk to inpatient health care facilities in California and identify regions at high risk.

METHODS

The California Department of Health and Human Services provides location and capacity information for all 15 684 licensed and certified health care facilities in California. In this study, we analyzed data updated as of October 2022 for licensed inpatient facilities, which treat patients for longer than 24 hours and may have complex evacuation needs.

The California Department of Forestry and Fire Protection (CAL FIRE) Fire and Resource Assessment Program classifies the state into 6 ordinal fire threat zone (FTZ) categories: not mapped, low, moderate, high, very high, and extreme. The threat zones "combine expected fire frequency with potential fire behavior," representing "the relative likelihood of damaging or difficult to control wildfires occurring for a given area."[6] As defined by CAL FIRE, the zones "can be used to assess the potential for impacts on various assets and values susceptible to fire[, and] impacts are more likely to occur and/or be of increased severity for the higher threat classes."[6]

Digital rasters representing fire threat obtained from CAL FIRE were converted to polygons at a 270-meter resolution, and nearest neighbor analyses were used to compute the distance from each facility to the nearest high, very high, or extreme FTZ.[7] Facilities within FTZs were assigned a distance of zero. The bed capacity for each facility was used to compute the distance of inpatient beds from each FTZ level.

We used Excel (Microsoft Corporation, Redmond, WA), QGIS version 3.16.7 (Open Source Geospatial Foundation, Beaverton, OR), and Python version 3.8 (Python Software Foundation, Wilmington, DE) in our analyses. All codes and underlying data are provided in Appendixes A through D (available as supplements to the online version of this article at http://www.ajph.org).

RESULTS

We included a total capacity of 214 358 inpatient beds (across 3087 inpatient facilities) in our analyses: 74 041 general and acute care beds at 429 facilities, 8961 beds at 135 behavioral health facilities, and 131 356 long-term care beds at 2523 facilities. Our results showed that 4 facilities are within a very high FTZ and 22 are within a high FTZ; 50% of total inpatient capacity (107 290 beds) is within 0.87 miles of a high FTZ (Figure 1), and 95% of capacity (203 665 beds) is within 3.7 miles of a high FTZ. In addition, half of the total inpatient bed capacity is within 3.3 miles of a very high FTZ and 15.5 miles of an extreme FTZ.

Median distance to an FTZ varies by county. The state's northern counties are disproportionately affected: there is lower overall capacity in these counties, and the median distances to high, very high, and extreme FTZs are substantially shorter. In the southern half of the state, San Luis Obispo County has the most inpatient facilities that are near FTZs (Appendixes B and C).

DISCUSSION

Wildfires in California can be rapid-onset disasters with a short preimpact or warning phase. This has left health care facility leadership and emergency preparedness specialists the option of either preparing hospitals for rapid evacuations or investing in adaptations that will allow hospital staff and patients to shelter in place until the wildfire no longer poses a threat.

Even if a facility is not under immediate threat of structural damage, smoke exposure, road closures, and infrastructure damage from nearby wildfires can have a longitudinal impact on health care system functioning and access to care.[8]

We found that a high percentage of inpatient health care facilities in California are at risk for potential operational disruption or evacuation from wildfires. Facilities near wildfires may face risks from windblown embers, transportation interruptions, and conversion of wildland fires to structure fires, which can affect the safety, operability, or accessibility of facilities or increase the risk of fire at facility sites.

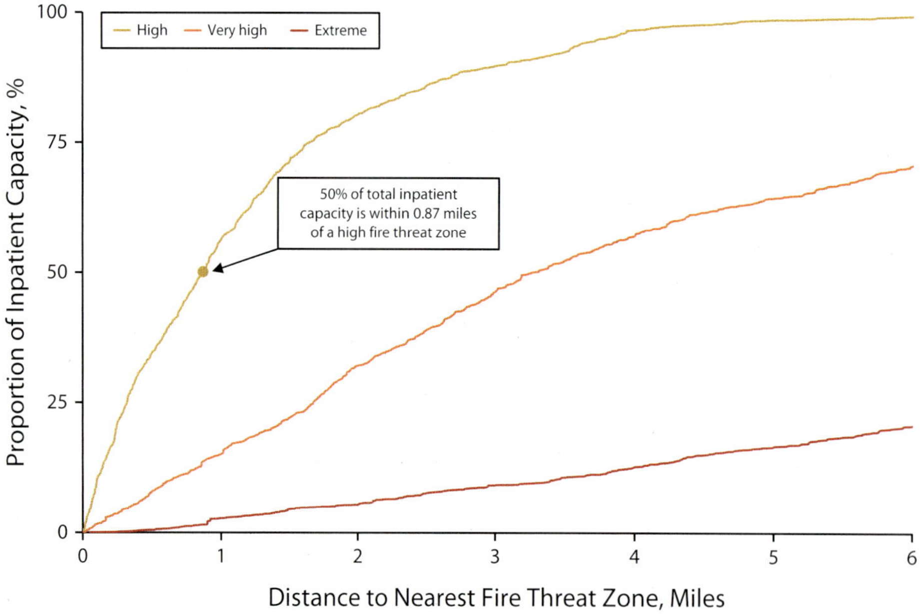

FIGURE 1— Distance of Inpatient Facilities From Fire Threat Zones: California, 2022

Note. The vertical axis represents the total inpatient capacity across the 3087 study facilities. The horizontal axis represents the distance from each facility to the nearest fire threat zone. Further methodological details are available in the Appendixes, available as a supplement to the online version of this article at http://www.ajph.org.

In northern counties—where 2 of California's largest fires burned more than 1 million acres over the past 2 years—health care accessibility is a significant concern because of high levels of hazard exposure and limited numbers of beds and facilities.

The large number of facilities at risk (despite representing a small proportion of total facilities) creates the possibility of complex evacuation needs as a result of the many potential sending and receiving facilities in a major fire scenario.

Limitations

The information on fire risk exposure reported here is based on CAL FIRE data and as such reflects current risk estimates.[6] Future fire risk in various climate change scenarios was not assessed and is expected to exceed current risk levels in many locations. Fire occurrence, propagation, and overall risk is a complex issue involving numerous dynamic variables. CAL FIRE FTZs are believed to be the best available source on which to base an analysis of such factors.

We did not attempt to assess or compare structural characteristics that could improve fire resistance or the degree of fire protection afforded by small-scale geographic features such as impervious surfaces and nonvegetated areas in health facilities' immediate environment, nor did we consider features that contribute to facility-level resilience such as backup generators and on-site fire suppression capabilities. Caution should be exercised when interpreting negative results; although a facility may not be near an FTZ or an active fire, facility operations may nonetheless be affected.

Public Health Implications

Our findings demonstrate widespread wildfire risk to inpatient health care facilities, including threats to much of the inpatient bed capacity in California. General hospitals are of particular concern because of difficulties associated with evacuation of hospitalized patients, limited numbers of alternate facilities to which patients can be evacuated, and the potential for loss of access to emergency care that accompanies even temporary closure of facilities.[9] The long-term care facility patient population is at high risk during evacuation; previous research demonstrates increased mortality during and after nursing home evacuations.[10] Involuntarily hospitalized patients in behavioral health facilities have special security needs during wildfire contingencies, making evacuation a complex undertaking.

We urge health facility leaders to assess the vulnerability of facilities to wildfire hazards and to prepare for both sheltering-in-place and evacuation scenarios. If sheltering patients and community evacuees is necessary, facilities must be prepared to optimize and allocate resources and have measures in place to mitigate the risk of wildfire smoke exposure. Health care facilities also should prepare for evacuation scenarios in which emergency medical services and patient transport resource availability may be scarce and access routes may be affected.[11]

The interinstitutional, transjurisdictional coordination and cooperation that will be required to minimize health care interruptions will necessitate investments in data architecture, community awareness, and infrastructure resilience.[12] Priorities may vary from region to region, reflecting differing regional risk profiles. As the climate crisis continues to raise wildfire risk, it is vital to protect inpatient health care facilities so that they can meet the needs of their communities.

AJPH

ABOUT THE AUTHORS

Neil Singh Bedi is with the Boston University School of Medicine, Boston, MA. Caleb Dresser and Satchit Balsari are with the Beth Israel Deaconess Medical Center/Harvard Medical School, Boston. Akash Yadav is with the Department of Epidemiology, Harvard University T. H. Chan School of Public Health, Boston. Andrew Schroeder is with Direct Relief, Santa Barbara, CA.

CORRESPONDENCE

Correspondence should be sent to Satchit Balsari, MD, MPH, 703C FXB Center for Health and Human Rights, 651 Huntington Ave, Boston, MA 02115 (e-mail: sbalsari@bidmc.harvard.edu). Reprints can be ordered at http://www.ajph.org by clicking the "Reprints" link.

PUBLICATION INFORMATION

Full Citation: Bedi NS, Dresser C, Yadav A, Schroeder A, Balsari S. Wildfire threat to inpatient health care facilities in California, 2022. *Am J Public Health*. 2023; 113(5):555–558.

Acceptance Date: January 14, 2023.

DOI: https://doi.org/10.2105/AJPH.2023.307236

CONTRIBUTORS

N. S. Bedi and C. Dresser conceived and designed the project, collected and analyzed data, and led the writing process. A. Yadav supported the conception and design and contributed significantly to analysis of the data. A. Schroeder and S. Balsari supported the project throughout, providing leadership, insight, and resources, and contributed significantly to the writing process.

ACKNOWLEDGMENTS

This work was supported by CrisisReady, a research collaboration at Harvard and Direct Relief funded in part by Google.org.

N. S. Bedi gives special thanks to his mentors and colleagues at CrisisReady and those within the climate and health community for their continuous guidance and support.

CONFLICTS OF INTEREST

All authors declare no competing interests.

HUMAN PARTICIPANT PROTECTION

Publicly accessible data were used in this study. No human participants were involved.

REFERENCES

1. California Department of Forestry and Fire Protection. Top 20 largest California wildfires. Available at: https://www.fire.ca.gov/media/4jandlhh/top20_acres.pdf. Accessed June 6, 2022.
2. Mace SE, Sharma A. Hospital evacuations due to disasters in the United States in the twenty-first century. *Am J Disaster Med.* 2020;15(1):7–22. https://doi.org/10.5055/ajdm.2020.0351
3. Ho C. The St. Helena hospital evacuated twice in five weeks due to California wildfires. Available at: https://www.sfchronicle.com/california-wildfires/article/The-St-Helena-hospital-that-evacuated-twice-in-15607257.php. Accessed June 1, 2022.
4. Sutherland S. 135 minutes. Available at: https://www.nfpa.org/News-and-Research/Publications-and-Media/NFPA-Journal/2019/January-February-2019/POV/Perspectives. Accessed June 1, 2022.
5. Adalja AA, Watson M, Bouri N, Minton K, Morhard RC, Toner ES. Absorbing citywide patient surge during Hurricane Sandy: a case study in accommodating multiple hospital evacuations. *Ann Emerg Med.* 2014;64(1):66–73.e1. https://doi.org/10.1016/j.annemergmed.2013.12.010
6. State of California and California Department of Forestry and Fire Protection. Fire threat map. Available at: https://frap.fire.ca.gov/media/10315/firethreat_19_ada.pdf. Accessed June 1, 2022.
7. Tenkanen H, Heikinheimo V. Nearest neighbor analysis with large data sets. Available at: https://autogis-site.readthedocs.io/en/2019/notebooks/L3/nearest-neighbor-faster.html. Accessed June 1, 2022.
8. Rosenthal A, Stover E, Haar RJ. Health and social impacts of California wildfires and the deficiencies in current recovery resources: an exploratory qualitative study of systems-level issues. *PLoS One.* 2021;16(3):e0248617. https://doi.org/10.1371/journal.pone.0248617
9. Hamideh S, Sen P, Fischer E. Wildfire impacts on education and healthcare: Paradise, California, after the Camp Fire. *Nat Hazards (Dordr).* 2022;111(1):353–387. https://doi.org/10.1007/s11069-021-05057-1
10. Dosa D, Feng Z, Hyer K, Brown LM, Thomas K, Mor V. Effects of Hurricane Katrina on nursing facility resident mortality, hospitalization, and functional decline. *Disaster Med Public Health Prep.* 2010;4(suppl 1):S28–S32. https://doi.org/10.1001/dmp.2010.11
11. Hassan EM, Mahmoud HN. Orchestrating performance of healthcare networks subjected to the compound events of natural disasters and pandemic. *Nat Commun.* 2021;12(1):1338. https://doi.org/10.1038/s41467-021-21581-x
12. Balsari S, Kiang MV, Buckee CO. Data in crisis—rethinking disaster preparedness in the United States. *N Engl J Med.* 2021;385(16):1526–1530. https://doi.org/10.1056/NEJMms2104654

Planning to Reduce the Health Impacts of Extreme Heat: A Content Analysis of Heat Action Plans in Local United States Jurisdictions

Juliette M. Randazza, MPH, MPA, Jeremy J. Hess, MD, MPH, Ann Bostrom, PhD, MBA, Cat Hartwell, MPH, Quinn H. Adams, MS, Amruta Nori-Sarma, PhD, MPH, Keith R. Spangler, PhD, ScM, Yuantong Sun, MS, Kate R. Weinberger, PhD, MA, Gregory A. Wellenius, ScD, MSc, and Nicole A. Errett, PhD, MSPH

See also Guardaro, p. 465.

Objectives. To examine commonalities and gaps in the content of local US heat action plans (HAPs) designed to decrease the adverse health effects of extreme heat.

Methods. We used content analysis to identify common strategies and gaps in extreme heat preparedness among written HAPs in the United States from jurisdictions that serve municipalities with more than 200 000 residents. We reviewed, coded, and analyzed plans to assess the prevalence of key components and strategies.

Results. All 21 plans evaluated incorporated data on activation triggers, heat health messaging and risk communication, cooling centers, surveillance activities, and agency coordination, and 95% incorporated information on outreach to at-risk populations. Gaps existed in the specific applications of these broad strategies.

Conclusions. Practice-based recommendations as well as future areas of research should focus on increasing targeted strategies for at-risk individuals and expanding the use of surveillance data outside of situational awareness. (*Am J Public Health.* 2023;113(5):559–567. https://doi.org/10.2105/AJPH.2022.307217)

AJPH May 2023, Vol 113, No. 5

As many regions in the United States experience increases in average temperatures attributable to climate change, extreme heat events have increased in frequency and duration.[1,2] Heat is a hazard that can combine with other environmental factors such as ozone and humidity to have catastrophic public health consequences.[3,4] Exposure to high heat is associated with increased emergency department visits, hospital admissions, and mortality rates and is tied to exacerbations of chronic conditions such as heart disease, stroke, diabetes, and acute renal failure.[5–7] From May to September each year, an average of 65 000 US residents visit emergency departments for heat exhaustion and heat stroke.[8] The Centers for Disease Control and Prevention (CDC) estimates that from 2004 to 2018 there were 10 527 deaths attributable to heat, approximately 702 deaths annually.[9] Heat-related illness, emergency department visits, and deaths are likely underestimated, with data missing on cases in which health conditions exacerbated by heat are attributed to another cause (e.g., cardiovascular disease).[8,10–12]

Studies involving other methods of estimation have produced mortality results much higher than CDC estimates.[11,12] For example, Shindell et al. estimated 12 000 heat-related deaths annually (95% confidence interval [CI] = 7400, 16 500), and Weinberger et al. estimated 5608 deaths annually (95% CI = 4748, 6291) in the contiguous United States.[11,12]

High heat has differing population and location effects. For example, 1 US study showed that heat-related deaths were highest among males, older adults, non-Hispanic Blacks, American

Indians/Alaska Natives, and those living in large metropolitan counties where the urban heat island effect (in which cities experience higher temperatures than surrounding rural areas as a result of building materials, air pollution, traffic, and decreased vegetation) is strongest.[9,13] Others most at risk include young children and people who are socially isolated, unhoused, working outdoors, or experiencing mental, cognitive, or other chronic illnesses.[8]

Heat action plans (HAPs) are written documents that help manage actions across multiple organizations to reduce adverse health effects from extreme heat. HAPs broadly contain strategies such as performing surveillance, providing risk communication, supporting social and health care, establishing cooling centers, distributing water bottles and fans, and creating energy assistance programs.[10,14] The geographic scope, timing, content, and participating organizations vary and depend on factors such as the partners involved in creation and implementation, capacity and resources available to lead agencies, and the populations within service areas. HAPs may decrease heat-related mortality to varying extents, although further research on evaluation and implementation is needed.[15–17] Often a component of HAPs, heatwave early warning systems provide alerts on heat risk and preventive actions and are activated by forecasted temperatures or other weather conditions.[14,18,19]

To our knowledge, there has not been a systematic assessment of the content of local US HAPs since 2004, including response strategies and their alignment with evidence-informed practice.[20] In response, we assessed the content of HAPs in large US cities and counties.

METHODS

Leveraging previous extreme heat response research and CDC-released guidance on core components of HAPs (specifically a report that combined findings from the literature and case studies on extreme heat response), we adapted legal assessment techniques to explore the content of US local HAPs.[10] Specific components recommended by the CDC include activation threshold, health data use, identification of vulnerable populations, monitoring and evaluation, and plan updates.[10] Potential interventions include surveillance, messaging and communications, social care and front-line health, cooling centers, water bottle distribution, fan distribution, energy assistance, changes to the built environment, and workplace heat alert programs.[10]

Study Population

We included municipalities with more than 200 000 residents according to the US Census Bureau's 2019 Annual Estimates of the Resident Population for Incorporated Places.[21] To obtain HAPs, we conducted a Web search, targeted outreach to local health departments and offices of emergency management (OEMs), and used plans previously obtained by journalists for their own research.[22] In total, 117 municipalities with an estimated population of 68 million people (20% of the US population) were included.[21] We identified 99 unique jurisdictions for inclusion as a result of instances in which county-level OEMs and public health agencies serve multiple jurisdictions. Our focus was informed by previous research identifying larger municipalities as more likely to have developed HAPs as a result of their size and available resources.[23]

Heat Action Plan Collection

An initial sample of HAPs from a journalistic source was supplemented with plans obtained directly from agencies.[22] We conducted Web searches for HAPs in jurisdictions with more than 200 000 residents using keywords such as "extreme heat," "heatwave," "heat action plan," "heat early warning system," "heat adaptation," and "public health heatwave management" in addition to local health department, OEM, jurisdiction, county, or city name. Also, we conducted searches for documents posted on agency Web sites by using the sites' search functions and the keywords just described. We then searched linked Web pages for downloadable plans. This strategy did not produce any downloadable plans but did inform the initial sampling frame for surveying agencies about their HAPs.

We conducted outreach as part of a national electronic survey that was active from September 2021 to January 2022. Surveys were sent to e-mail addresses of representatives (including emergency management directors, health directors or officers, and environmental health or public health preparedness coordinators) at local health departments and OEMs obtained from agency Web sites or from follow-up telephone calls to agencies. Although multiple representatives for each jurisdiction were contacted, they were asked to coordinate responses. In total, we sent 4 reminder e-mails beyond the initial contact e-mail and extended the active survey window to incorporate further responses.

We collected survey data using the online electronic data collection software

REDCap (Research Electronic Data Capture). As part of the survey, jurisdictions were asked whether they had a written HAP, policy, or procedure and were asked to upload their most recently updated document (or documents).

Inclusion and Exclusion

Inclusion criteria for documents were as follows: standalone HAPs, standard operating procedures, checklists, protocols, or annexes to emergency or hazard mitigation plans used for extreme heat emergencies. Also, HAPs had to have been created or updated since 2016. HAPs were excluded if they were (1) emergency or hazard mitigation plans that did not include specific actions to address extreme heat preparedness and response during heat emergencies or (2) plans that did not address response to acute heat emergencies but instead focused on long-term planning.

Analysis

We adapted legal assessment and qualitative content analysis techniques and systematically applied categorical classification by coding the plan text and using the coded text to answer specific questions.[24] Codebook development proceeded through a combination of methods. Components of HAPs identified by the CDC and previous research on county-level heat preparedness and response were used to develop the analytical framework and preliminary set of codes through deductive methods.[10,23] After review of a sample of plans, we inductively developed additional codes to identify parts of plans that deductive codes were not able to capture (e.g., whether cooling center locations are predetermined or established ad hoc during emergencies), as well as corresponding coding questions.[25,26]

Codes included definitions and directions for use (Appendix A, available as a supplement to the online version of this article at http://www.ajph.org). We developed coding questions in binary or categorical formats and linked them to specific codes (Figure 1 and Appendix B, available as a supplement to the online version of this article at http://www.ajph.org). We documented revisions to codes and used NVivo for PC software (QSR International, Burlington, MA) to code HAPs. When there was ambiguity or nuance, records of the coder's decisions were logged. Ten percent of HAPs were co-coded by 2 investigators (J. M. R. and a non-author collaborator) independently, and results were compared and evaluated for discrepancies to refine code definitions and provide examples of application.[25] J. M. R. coded the remainder of plans. We recorded answers to coding questions in a Microsoft Excel database and synthesized code content to illustrate common strategies and gaps in plans.[27]

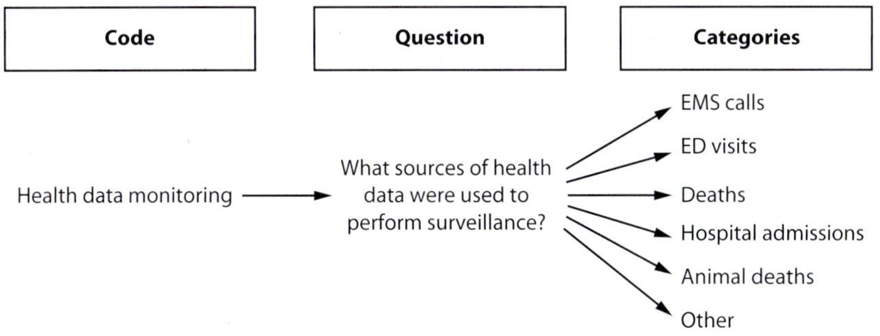

FIGURE 1— Codes, Corresponding Coding Questions, and Categories of Data Obtained From Coding Questions for Analysis of US Heat Action Plans

Note. ED = emergency department; EMS = emergency medical service.

RESULTS

We obtained and analyzed 21 plans, 9 (42.9%) from previous journalistic research and 12 (57.1%) from our survey responses. The jurisdictional populations covered by these plans ranged from 321 793 to 8 467 000, with a median of 967 640 people. We did not identify additional plans after conducting Web searches. Of the analyzed plans, 14 (66.7%) were standalone or separate from larger all-hazards plans, and 17 (81.0%) listed an OEM as lead or co-lead of plan administration. Although public health agencies had a role in the implementation of all plans, only 6 (28.6%) plans listed them as the lead or co-lead.

Seven of the 10 US Department of Health and Human Services administrative regions were represented in our analysis (Figure 2). Table 1 displays an overview of the different types of strategies and the numbers and percentages of plans that addressed the strategies.

Plan Activation, Scaling, and Termination

Twenty plans (95.2%) used National Weather Service (NWS) advisories as triggers for plan activation, with 7 of these plans (35.0%) using NWS alerts as the sole trigger. Other plans combined alerts with triggers such as epidemiological surveillance thresholds

AJPH May 2023, Vol 113, No. 5

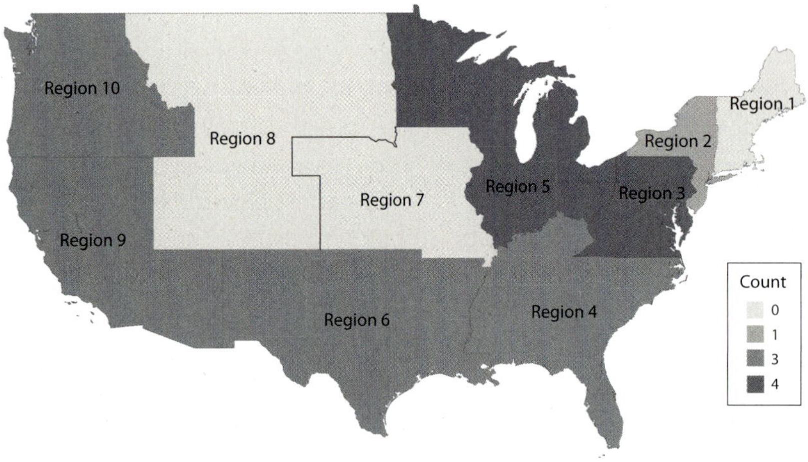

FIGURE 2— Geographical Distribution of Analyzed Heat Action Plans by US Department of Health and Human Services Region: United States, 2016–2021

linked to deaths or heat illness, the heat index independent of NWS alerts, ongoing infrastructure effects such as rolling blackouts, stakeholder requests, and abnormal livestock mortality rates. Seventeen plans (81.0%) also included definitions relevant to heat waves such as heat index, extreme heat, heat advisory, excessive heat warning or watch, excessive heat outlook, and heat-related mortality. The NWS was the source of most definitions (71.4%).

Seventeen plans (81.0%) incorporated scaled responses in which different levels of agency response were triggered seasonally or according to heat event severity. For example, date-based triggers were used to commence early season risk communication strategies and epidemiological surveillance. Extreme high heat indexes were used in triggering activation of emergency operations centers to coordinate interagency responses, whereas lower heat indexes were in some instances used in triggering smaller-scale situational awareness activities between agencies.

Eight plans (38.1%) described response deescalation through either specific thresholds (e.g., expiration or cancellation of heat advisories or warnings from the NWS) or deactivation activities such as termination alerts to participating organizations and agencies.

Risk Communication

All plans included strategies for communicating risks associated with extreme heat to the public. Recipients of information on specific communication strategies included at-risk populations (71.4%), community-based organizations (33.3%), government agency staff members (33.3%), social and case workers (14.3%), schools and day-care centers (14.3%), health care providers (14.3%), and first responders (9.5%). Message content included alerts and warnings, heat safety tips, encouragement to "check in with your neighbor," reminders to conserve power, and

TABLE 1— Heat Action Plans That Included Heat Action Strategies: United States, 2016–2021

Strategy	% (No.)	DHHS Regions With Strategy Performed
Risk communication	100.0 (21)	All regions represented in study
Surveillance and monitoring	100.0 (21)	All regions represented in study
Interagency and interorganizational coordination	100.0 (21)	All regions represented in study
Cooling centers	100.0 (21)	All regions represented in study
Targeted outreach to at-risk populations	95.2 (20)	All regions represented in study
Scaled response	81.0 (17)	All regions represented in study
Social care interventions	66.7 (14)	All regions represented in study
Update and review	66.7 (14)	3, 4, 5, 6, 9, 10
Cooling shelters	48.0 (10)	3, 4, 5, 6, 9
Health interventions	43.0 (9)	3, 4, 5, 6, 10
Plan termination	38.1 (8)	3, 4, 6, 9, 10

Note. DHHS = Department of Health and Human Services. See Figure 2 for region numbers.

information on service provisions such as the locations of cooling centers.

Eighteen plans (85.7%) listed the intended communication platforms for message dissemination. The most common forms of communication were traditional media sources such as radio and television, call centers, government agency Web sites, emergency alert systems, and social media.

Seven plans (33.3%) included strategies promoting language accessibility in communication materials. Common strategies included creating outreach materials in Spanish or multiple languages, providing closed captioning or sign language for press releases, and releasing alerts in plain language or accessible formats according to agency guidelines.

Surveillance and Monitoring

All plans detailed surveillance or monitoring. In the case of 2 plans, however, this was restricted to monitoring weather forecasts and NWS notifications rather than collecting in-house data. Eighteen plans (85.7%) detailed health data collection, the most common forms of which were emergency department visits, deaths, hospital admissions, and emergency medical service calls. Sixteen plans (76.2%) explicitly described monitoring weather and other environmental data such as air quality and humidity through NWS or other forecasts. Ten plans (47.6%) included monitoring at-risk populations such as people using shelters or those experiencing houselessness, residents of skilled nursing and assisted living facilities, and people reliant on medical equipment. Plans also described collecting information on cooling center use, fire and police call volumes, and utility infrastructure conditions.

Surveillance and monitoring data were most often used for situational awareness (e.g., resource needs, event cancellations and modifications, energy infrastructure status, and demand on the health care system) during heat events. Data were used less frequently after heat events (e.g., in end-of-summer reporting, heat response reviews, and damage assessments) or to track health trends over time.

Agency Coordination

All plans described coordination between lead agencies and supporting government agencies (at the city, county, state, and federal levels) and between lead agencies and nongovernmental and private organizations. To manage coordination between agencies and jurisdictions, 16 plans (76.2%) incorporated incident response structures (e.g., the National Incident Management System) or activation of an emergency operations center. Coordination strategies included developing situation reports and hosting briefings, organizing task forces, preestablishing points of contact, holding annual preseason stakeholder meetings, and using WebEOC or other emergency management software to share information. Coordination strategies created opportunities for situational awareness, provision of agency-specific data and identification of concerns, organization of planning efforts for response and recovery, and management of resource and mutual aid requests between different organizations, agencies, and levels of government.

Descriptions of coordination between agencies and nongovernmental, private, and faith-based organizations involved multidirectional information exchange. Plans indicated that agencies would provide alerts and updates at the beginning of and during heat emergencies, whereas nongovernmental organizations were often described as sources of information for monitoring at-risk populations. Nongovernmental organizations were also described as providing services such as staffing cooling centers and conducting well-being checks. These activities required communicating resource needs and updates to emergency and public health agencies. Plans described other opportunities for coordination as well, such as development of organizational response plans, inclusion of organizational representatives in task forces and planning activities, and amplification of communication efforts.

Cooling Centers and Shelters

All plans included descriptions of cooling center or shelter implementation. Cooling shelters, meant for overnight stays and most often intended for people experiencing houselessness, were described separately from cooling centers, with some plans providing specific definitions for each. Ten (47.6%) plans referenced cooling shelter strategies such as predetermined locations and transportation to sites.

Implementation considerations for cooling centers included resources such as water, seating, and first aid as well as operational considerations such as staffing and finding locations accessible for people with access or functional needs. Two thirds (66.7%) of plans incorporated strategies to provide access to transportation to cooling centers or shelters. These strategies included waiving transit fees to cooling centers and providing transportation to specific populations such as those experiencing houselessness, older adults, and people with access or functional needs.

Plans described predetermined locations (42.9%), ad hoc locations (42.9%), or a combination of both (9.5%) or did not specify locations (4.7%) for cooling centers or shelters. Common locations included senior centers, recreation and community centers, buses, libraries, jurisdictional facilities, faith-based or nonprofit-operated facilities, shopping malls, movie theaters, restaurants, and park facilities such as pools and spray parks.

Health and Social Care

Ten plans (47.6%) described health system–related interventions such as creating mobile hospitals and clinics, providing first aid and triage at cooling centers and cooling buses, stocking appropriate medical supplies for field personnel, providing spiritual and emotional care, requesting additional emergency medical service system capacity, and communicating risks to health care personnel and first responders. Fourteen plans (66.7%) included strategies for well-being and in-home checks from community-based organizations, social workers, and other providers.

Targeted Outreach

All plans identified specific populations most at risk for effects of extreme heat. Twenty plans (95.2%) detailed specific outreach and communication strategies for people at risk, with 16 (76.2%) including 1 or more general outreach strategies to "at-risk populations" without specifying populations or individuals and 15 (71.4%) including 1 or more outreach strategies to specific populations or individuals (Figure 3).

General strategies included partnerships with organizations for communicating risks, identifying at-risk populations, conducting well-being checks, and providing transportation or evacuation to cooling centers and shelters. Specific strategies included water distribution, financial assistance, building inspections, modification of athletic events, and coordination with school districts.

Although 5 plans (23.8%) explicitly identified low-income residents as at risk for heat effects, only 1 incorporated financial assistance programs. Seven plans did not identify low-income residents as at risk but included financial assistance programs such as utility moratoriums, utility assistance, and fan or air conditioner distribution.

Update and Review

Fourteen plans (66.7%) described processes for update and review such as conducting updates (61.9%), providing staff or responder training (28.6%), and conducting postevent reviews (28.6%). One plan incorporated all these processes and 9 incorporated 2 of the processes. Timing varied among the plans that included update procedures, with about half occurring annually (53.8%) and others occurring every 2 years (7.7%), every 3 years (7.7%), after an event (23.0%), or at an unspecified point (30.8%). In 3 plans (23.0%), updates were performed after both a specific number of years and an event. Postevent reviews occurred as after-action discussions (e.g., hot washes), reports, and improvement plans. Four of the plans (66.7%) that did include postevent reviews specified incorporation of surveillance data into review processes.

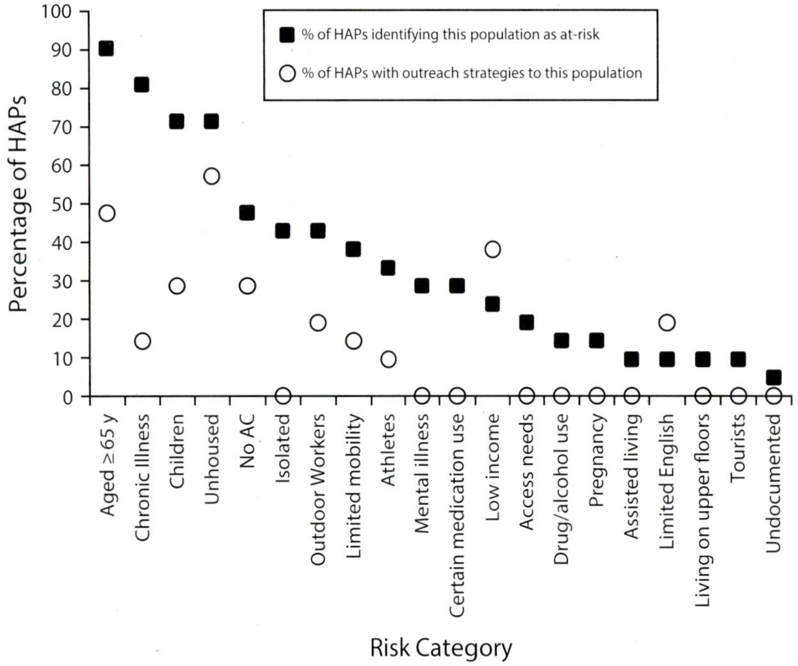

FIGURE 3— Percentage of Populations Identified as At-Risk in Heat Action Plans (HAPs) Compared With Percentage of Populations Targeted Through Specific HAP Outreach Strategies: United States, 2016–2021

Note. AC = air conditioning.

DISCUSSION

As heat waves threaten the health and well-being of residents in many regions of the United States, HAPs at the local level can bridge gaps between research and practice by incorporating evidence-informed strategies and play a key role in guiding multiorganizational responses during extreme heat emergencies. The HAPs reviewed in this study included many recommendations from previous research on heat response as well as CDC guidance.

Most, if not all, plans identified a lead agency, provided activation triggers, and described strategies for heat health messaging and risk communication, cooling centers, surveillance activities, at-risk population outreach, and agency coordination. Although plans incorporated most major categories of strategies, applications and inclusion of implementation and evaluation components varied. All plans identified specific at-risk populations, the most common of whom were older adults, people living with acute or chronic illness, infants and children, and people experiencing houselessness. Strategies that included specific at-risk populations were most often aimed at older adults or those experiencing houselessness.

As demonstrated in Figure 3, gaps exist between populations considered at risk by the plans and specific outreach to these populations. In addition, given that other populations are also at risk for extreme heat, opportunities exist for increased outreach and dissemination of communications to these populations. For example, only 2 plans described communication to health care providers, who can act as trusted sources of information for patients and may provide targeted outreach to otherwise historically underserved people who have certain illnesses or use certain medications.[28] Although many plans incorporated varied platforms for risk communication, only 33% included language accessibility in their communication strategies and only 9.5% identified people with limited English proficiency as at risk for extreme heat, despite previous research indicating limited English proficiency as a risk factor for poor outcomes during disasters.[29]

Although all plans included strategies for surveillance and monitoring, few described use of the information derived from these activities to inform implementation or evaluation activities. The CDC recommends that epidemiological surveillance be used to determine people, places, and times of greatest risk.[10] Epidemiological data have also been used by academic institutions and jurisdictions in collaboration with the NWS to revise heat advisory levels.[30–32] These uses of surveillance data occur outside active emergency situations, yet current applications focus on immediate use for situational awareness. Use of surveillance data in planning and recovery efforts presents an opportunity to increase and bolster plan monitoring and evaluation, a neglected component of HAPs.

Notably absent in the analyzed HAPs were long-term planning strategies such as green roofs, parks, and green space and vegetation, which are recommended by the CDC and are linked to cooler city microclimates.[10] This may be a result of the emergency response focus of the analyzed plans and the exclusion of plans focused on longer-term mitigation.[33] Partnerships at the local level between OEMs and city planning and sustainability divisions, however, are an important component of long-term heat planning and should be prioritized. Additional research is necessary to explore integration of such longer-term strategies in hazard mitigation and climate adaptation plans.

Limitations

Our study included only plans available online or shared by jurisdictions. The COVID-19 pandemic likely limited the capacity of local health departments to respond to our survey and provide their HAPs. This convenience sampling approach limits the generalizability of our results in addition to precluding assessment of geographic differences in heat preparedness and response, which is an important area for future research. Notably, key strategies and gaps identified in our analysis were from plans of large, well-resourced jurisdictions expected to be furthest in plan development. Furthermore, cities that provided plans may have been more advanced in their planning than those that did not.

Also, the plans included in our study may not be the most recent or inclusive of all heat adaptation activities within a given jurisdiction. In addition, we were unable to determine the extent to which plans were implemented. Plan implementation and population health effects are areas for future research. Finally, plans that were not specific to heat, such as comprehensive emergency management plans, were excluded. Strategies outlined in comprehensive emergency management plans, such as mass care, may have application in heat emergencies but were excluded because the conditions and extent to which these strategies would be employed during a heat emergency were not apparent.

Public Health Implications

HAPs are policy tools that engage multiple stakeholders in extreme heat planning and can help guide responses during heat emergencies, potentially reducing the morbidity and mortality associated with these events. This study provides insight into current strategies and gaps in jurisdictional extreme heat planning in the United States. Although many plans incorporate components identified by research and government guidance, opportunities exist to increase language accessibility, implement strategies targeted to specific at-risk groups, and incorporate surveillance into planning. Responsive plan updates can be supported through agency and organizational partnerships, development of new guidance and templates, and technical assistance. AJPH

ABOUT THE AUTHORS

At the time of the study, Juliette M. Randazza was with the Department of Environmental and Occupational Health Sciences, School of Public Health, University of Washington, Seattle. Jeremy J. Hess is with the Departments of Global Health and Environmental and Occupational Health Sciences, School of Public Health, and the Department of Emergency Medicine, School of Medicine, University of Washington. Ann Bostrom is with the Daniel J. Evans School of Public Policy and Governance, University of Washington. Cat Hartwell and Nicole A. Errett are with the Department of Environmental and Occupational Health Sciences, School of Public Health, University of Washington. Quinn H. Adams, Amruta Nori-Sarma, Keith R. Spangler, Yuantong Sun, and Gregory A. Wellenius are with the Department of Environmental Health, School of Public Health, Boston University, Boston, MA. At the time of the study, Kate R. Weinberger was with the Occupational and Environmental Health Division, School of Population and Public Health, University of British Columbia, Vancouver, BC, Canada.

CORRESPONDENCE

Correspondence should be sent to Nicole A. Errett, PhD, MSPH, 4225 Roosevelt Way NE, Seattle, WA 98105 (e-mail: nerrett@uw.edu). Reprints can be ordered at http://www.ajph.org by clicking the "Reprints" link.

PUBLICATION INFORMATION

Full Citation: Randazza JM, Hess JJ, Bostrom A, et al. Planning to reduce the health impacts of extreme heat: a content analysis of heat action plans in local United States jurisdictions. *Am J Public Health*. 2023;113(5):559–567.

Acceptance Date: December 18, 2022.

DOI: https://doi.org/10.2105/AJPH.2022.307217

CONTRIBUTORS

J. M. Randazza, J. J. Hess, A. Bostrom, A. Nori Sarma, K. R. Weinberger, G. A. Wellenius, and N. A. Errett designed the research, with input from C. Hartwell, Q. H. Adams, K. R. Spangler, and Y. Sun. J. M. Randazza, C. Hartwell, and N. A. Errett contributed to the implementation of the research. J. M. Randazza, J. J. Hess, A. Bostrom, C. Hartwell, K. R. Spangler, K. R. Weinberger, G. A. Wellenius, and N. A. Errett contributed to the analysis of the results. All authors contributed to the interpretation of results and writing of the article.

ACKNOWLEDGMENTS

This project was supported by the Wellcome Trust (grant 216033-Z-19-Z).

We collected and managed study data using REDCap (Research Electronic Data Capture), which is hosted at the University of Washington's Institute of Translational Health Sciences and supported by the National Center for Advancing Translational Sciences of the National Institutes of Health (NIH) under award UL1 TR002319.

Special thanks to Joanne Medina for assistance in coding.

Note. The content is solely the responsibility of the authors and does not necessarily represent the official views of the NIH.

CONFLICTS OF INTEREST

G. A. Wellenius receives consulting income from the Health Effects Institute (Boston, MA) and Google LLC (Mountain View, CA). All other authors declare no competing interests.

HUMAN PARTICIPANT PROTECTION

No human participant data were gathered or reviewed. This study was determined not to be human participant research by the University of Washington's Human Subjects Division.

REFERENCES

1. Hayhoe K, Wuebbles DJ, Easterling DR, et al. Fourth National Climate Assessment: impacts, risks, and adaptation in the United States. Available at: https://nca2018.globalchange.gov. Accessed April 26, 2022.
2. Perkins-Kirkpatrick SE, Lewis SC. Increasing trends in regional heatwaves. *Nat Commun*. 2020;11(1):3357. https://doi.org/10.1038/s41467-020-16970-7
3. Filleul L, Cassadou S, Médina S, et al. The relation between temperature, ozone, and mortality in nine French cities during the heat wave of 2003. *Environ Health Perspect*. 2006;114(9):1344–1347. https://doi.org/10.1289/ehp.8328
4. Raymond C, Matthews T, Horton RM. The emergence of heat and humidity too severe for human tolerance. *Sci Adv*. 2020;6(19):eaaw1838. https://doi.org/10.1126/sciadv.aaw1838
5. Basu R, Pearson D, Malig B, Broadwin R, Green R. The effect of high ambient temperature on emergency room visits. *Epidemiology*. 2012;23(6):813–820. https://doi.org/10.1097/EDE.0b013e31826b7f97
6. Lugo-Amador NM, Rothenhaus T, Moyer P. Heat-related illness. *Emerg Med Clin North Am*. 2004;22(2):315–327. https://doi.org/10.1016/j.emc.2004.01.004
7. Anderson GB, Bell ML. Heat waves in the United States: mortality risk during heat waves and effect modification by heat wave characteristics in 43 US communities. *Environ Health Perspect*. 2011;119(2):210–218. https://doi.org/10.1289/ehp.1002313
8. US Global Change Research Program. Impacts of climate change on human health in the United States: a scientific assessment. Available at: https://health2016.globalchange.gov. Accessed April 26, 2022.
9. Vaidyanathan A, Malilay J, Schramm P, Saha S. Heat-related deaths—United States, 2004–2018. *MMWR Morb Mortal Wkly Rep*. 2020;69(24):729–734. https://doi.org/10.15585/mmwr.mm6924a1
10. US National Center for Environmental Health. Heat response plans: summary of evidence and strategies for collaboration and implementation. Available at: https://stacks.cdc.gov/view/cdc/93705. Accessed April 26, 2022.
11. Shindell D, Zhang Y, Scott M, Ru M, Stark K, Ebi KL. The effects of heat exposure on human mortality throughout the United States. *GeoHealth*. 2020;4(4):e2019GH000234. https://doi.org/10.1029/2019GH000234
12. Weinberger KR, Harris D, Spangler KR, Zanobetti A, Wellenius GA. Estimating the number of excess deaths attributable to heat in 297 United States counties. *Environ Epidemiol*. 2020;4(3):e096. https://doi.org/10.1097/EE9.0000000000000096
13. Kleerekoper L, Van Esch M, Salcedo TB. How to make a city climate-proof, addressing the urban heat island effect. *Resour Conserv Recycling*. 2012;64:30–38. https://doi.org/10.1016/j.resconrec.2011.06.004
14. Casanueva A, Burgstall A, Kotlarski S, et al. Overview of existing heat-health warning systems in Europe. *Int J Environ Res Public Health*. 2019;16(15):2657. https://doi.org/10.3390/ijerph16152657
15. Ebi KL, Teisberg TJ, Kalkstein LS, Robinson L, Weiher RF. Heat watch/warning systems save lives: estimated costs and benefits for Philadelphia 1995–1998. *Bull Am Meteorol Soc*. 2004;85(8):1067–1074. https://doi.org/10.1175/BAMS-85-8-1067
16. Boeckmann M, Rohn I. Is planned adaptation to heat reducing heat-related mortality and illness? A systematic review. *BMC Public Health*. 2014;14(1):1112. https://doi.org/10.1186/1471-2458-14-1112
17. Steul K, Schade M, Heudorf U. Mortality during heatwaves 2003–2015 in Frankfurt-Main—the 2003 heatwave and its implications. *Int J Hyg Environ Health*. 2018;221(1):81–86. https://doi.org/10.1016/j.ijheh.2017.10.005
18. Lowe D, Ebi KL, Forsberg B. Heatwave early warning systems and adaptation advice to reduce human health consequences of heatwaves. *Int J Environ Res Public Health*. 2011;8(12):4623–4648. https://doi.org/10.3390/ijerph8124623
19. Hajat S, Sheridan SC, Allen MJ, et al. Heat-health warning systems: a comparison of the predictive capacity of different approaches to identifying dangerously hot days. *Am J Public Health*. 2010;100(6):1137–1144. https://doi.org/10.2105/AJPH.2009.169748
20. Bernard SM, McGeehin MA. Municipal heat wave response plans. *Am J Public Health*. 2004;94(9):1520–1522. https://doi.org/10.2105/AJPH.94.9.1520

21. US Census Bureau. City and town population totals: 2010–2019. Available at: https://www.census.gov/data/tables/time-series/demo/popest/2010s-total-cities-and-towns.html. Accessed April 26, 2022.
22. Rock J, August H. Killer heat: US cities' plans for coming heatwaves fail to protect vulnerable. Available at: https://www.theguardian.com/cities/2019/dec/06/killer-heat-us-cities-plans-for-coming-heatwaves-fail-to-protect-vulnerable. Accessed April 28, 2021.
23. White-Newsome JL, Ekwurzel B, Baer-Schultz M, Ebi KL, O'Neill MS, Anderson GB. Survey of county-level heat preparedness and response to the 2011 summer heat in 30 US states. *Environ Health Perspect.* 2014;122(6):573–579. https://doi.org/10.1289/ehp.1306693
24. Cho JY, Lee EH. Reducing confusion about grounded theory and qualitative content analysis: similarities and differences. *Qual Rep.* 2014;19(32):1–20. https://doi.org/10.46743/2160-3715/2014.1028
25. Anderson ED, Tremper C, Thomas S, Wagenaar AC. Measuring statutory law and regulations for empirical research. Available at: https://phlr.org/sites/default/files/downloads/resource/MeasuringLawRegulationsforEmpiricalResearch-Monograph-AndersonTremper-March2012.pdf. Accessed April 28, 2021.
26. Thomas DR. A general inductive approach for analyzing qualitative evaluation data. *Am J Eval.* 2006;27(2):237–246. https://doi.org/10.1177/1098214005283748
27. Elo S, Kyngäs H. The qualitative content analysis process. *J Adv Nurs.* 2008;62(1):107–115. https://doi.org/10.1111/j.1365-2648.2007.04569.x
28. Brodie M, Kjellson N, Hoff T, Parker M. Perceptions of Latinos, African Americans, and whites on media as a health information source. *Howard J Commun.* 1999;10(3):147–167. https://doi.org/10.1080/106461799246799
29. Thomas DS, Phillips BD, Fothergill A, Blinn-Pike L. *Social Vulnerability to Disasters.* Boca Raton, FL: CRC Press; 2009.
30. Wellenius GA, Eliot MN, Bush KF, et al. Heat-related morbidity and mortality in New England: evidence for local policy. *Environ Res.* 2017;156:845–853. https://doi.org/10.1016/j.envres.2017.02.005
31. Adeyeye TE, Insaf TZ, Al-Hamdan MZ, et al. Estimating policy-relevant health effects of ambient heat exposures using spatially contiguous reanalysis data. *Environ Health.* 2019;18(1):35. https://doi.org/10.1186/s12940-019-0467-5
32. Insaf T, Estes MG Jr, Adeyeye TE, et al. Heat warning decision support system enhancements in New York State using satellite derived estimates of air temperature. Available at: https://ui.adsabs.harvard.edu/abs/2018AGUFMGH34B..02I/abstract. Accessed April 28, 2021.
33. US Environmental Protection Agency. Reduce urban heat island effect. Available at: https://www.epa.gov/green-infrastructure/reduce-urban-heat-island-effect. Accessed May 23, 2022.

Loopholes for Underage Access in E-Cigarette Delivery Sales Laws, United States, 2022

Sunday Azagba, PhD, Todd Ebling, PhD, Olayemi Timothy Adekeye, MPS, Mark Hall, JD, and Jessica King Jensen, PhD

See also Gottlieb, p. 472.

Objectives. To comprehensively catalog and review state e-cigarette delivery sales laws as well as capture their scope and dimensions.

Methods. We conducted an in-depth review to determine whether states had at least 1 form of e-cigarette delivery sales law. We coded laws for 5 key policy domains: (1) delivery terminology used in laws, (2) age verification requirements, (3) packaging label requirements, (4) permit or registration requirements, and (5) fines and penalties for violations.

Results. Overall, 34 states had e-cigarette delivery sales laws with varying scopes and dimensions. In 27 states, these laws required at least 1 form of age verification requirements. We identified mandatory packaging labels in 12 states, and 7 states where permits were required. There were considerable differences among states on the scale of fines and penalties for violations.

Conclusions. Our findings reveal extensive heterogeneity in e-cigarette delivery sales laws among states, particularly regarding the scope and dimensions of these laws.

Public Health Implications. The mapping of e-cigarette delivery sales policies showed several potential loopholes that may diminish their effectiveness. (*Am J Public Health*. 2023;113(5):568–576. https://doi.org/10.2105/AJPH.2023.307228)

AJPH May 2023, Vol 113, No. 5

For more than 2 decades, the Internet has created numerous challenges to governing the remote sale of tobacco products effectively.[1] One crucial issue for policymakers has been how to protect adolescents and youths from the harms of smoking, considering how few restrictions exist on online purchase and delivery.[2,3] In the absence of binding federal law, many states enacted delivery laws in the early 1990 s to mid-2000 s to restrict youth access to cigarettes.[4] However, since 2014, electronic cigarettes (e-cigarettes) have become the most used tobacco product by young people.[5] E-cigarettes now make up a multibillion-dollar industry, with high e-cigarette use rates among young people, including an estimated 2.55 million middle school and high school students as current users.[6] E-cigarette aerosol contains volatile organic compounds, ultrafine particles, heavy metals such as nickel and lead, and carcinogens, all potentially harmful to users.[7,8] E-cigarettes almost invariably contain nicotine, which can impair adolescent and young adult brain development and lead to long-term use.[7,9,10]

E-cigarette brands have targeted youths online, and app-based delivery services have made e-cigarettes more accessible to youths. E-cigarette product promotion is widespread among Internet vendors, and e-commerce sales make up a significant but hard-to-track marketplace for e-cigarettes.[11–13] An estimated 32% of adolescents reported ever purchasing a vape device online in 2016,[14] and 8%, or nearly 20 000 youths, reported usually purchasing e-cigarettes online.[15] Additionally, exploiting the limited in-person interaction caused by the COVID-19 pandemic, e-cigarette marketers aggressively encouraged customers to order e-cigarettes online and have the products delivered to their homes.[16] Despite the prevalence of e-cigarette e-commerce and its focused allure for youths,[17] many US states still do not have laws regulating or restricting e-cigarette sales delivery.

At the federal level, the Jenkins Act of 1949 and the Preventing All Cigarette Trafficking (PACT) Act of 2009 were amended by Congress in December 2020 through the enactment of the Preventing Online Sales of E-Cigarettes to Children Act. The Jenkins Act initially established tax-reporting requirements for vendors who shipped cigarettes across state lines, and the PACT Act required remote sellers of tobacco products to pay all applicable federal, state, and local taxes and comply with all applicable state and local laws. The new legislation amended the definition of "cigarette" to include "e-cigarette," defined as "any electronic device that, through an aerosolized solution, delivers nicotine, flavor, or any other substance to the user inhaling from the device."[18] Further, the 2020 act prohibits delivery vendors from using the US Postal Service to ship e-cigarettes, which applies to all interstate commerce shipments. Several other major carriers (e.g., United Parcel Service, FedEx, and DHL) have voluntarily followed suit to ban e-cigarette delivery through their services.[19] However, remote sellers of e-cigarettes have turned to alternative means of delivery, such as contracted drivers, to continue reaching this market segment.[20] The PACT Act also requires tobacco vendors to verify age and identity at purchase, to use a method of mailing or shipping that checks identification, and to label shipping packages as containing tobacco. However, prior studies have shown limited compliance with these practices.[13,21]

At the state level, various laws have been implemented to further regulate in-state e-cigarette sales and use.[22] A prominent concern for state policymakers is limiting youth access.[23] State delivery sales laws offer a promising opportunity to further diminish youth access to e-cigarettes, yet very little is known about the scope and dimensions of such laws. This study aimed to comprehensively catalog state e-cigarette delivery sales laws as well as capture their scope and dimensions. We reviewed and coded state laws in 2022 to shed light on this timely issue and provide a novel comprehensive review that could help inform effective decision-making in e-cigarette delivery sales laws.

METHODS

We drew baseline data from the Public Health Law Center (PHLC) e-cigarette regulation database.[24] The PHLC is a law school–based research institute that documents tobacco statutes and regulations that specify various key elements of these laws. We further assessed initial laws using Casetext and Westlaw, 2 online legal reference databases. We conducted an in-depth review of delivery sales statutes, along with more general state laws that were relevant. Anywhere primary statutes overtly referenced related statutes, we reviewed them to establish their significance and collected them if relevant to our study. Independently, at least 2 reviewers assessed, compiled, and analyzed state laws explicitly regulating e-cigarette delivery sales; discrepancies in coding or analysis were resolved through consensus. All laws were accessed, reviewed, and coded between July 1, 2022, and December 2, 2022. Specifically, we coded 5 key policy domains:

1. delivery terminology used in laws,
2. age verification requirements,
3. packaging label requirements,
4. permit or registration requirements, and
5. fines and penalties for violations.

Delivery Terminology Used in Laws

We coded the explicit delivery terminology used in the laws, focusing on the most regularly used terms: delivery, remote, Internet, mail, phone, voice, and fax (facsimile). Additionally, we captured terms commonly used in broader categories. For example, "Internet" also includes "electronic network," "computer network," and "online."

Age Verification Requirements

Reviewers captured whether laws required a form of age verification upon purchase or delivery of e-cigarette products. For age verification at purchase, we identified whether states required proof via a category we labeled "database." This category involved verifying a customer's identity and age by comparing their provided information with public records, a third-party database, or aggregate databases. The coded set "payment" identified states requiring payment only through a credit or debit card or a check written in the purchaser's name. The group "certification" recognized states requiring a form of certification in which the potential purchaser attests that they are of the legal age to make the purchase. We coded "Gov ID (P)" to indicate whether a valid form of government identification was required for delivery purchase and "Gov ID (D)" to indicate the same requirement for the release of the product at delivery. Lastly, we coded states requiring a signature by either an adult of legal e-cigarette purchasing age or by the specific purchaser of the e-cigarette product for release of the product at delivery.

Packaging Label Requirement

Coders indicated whether a specific delivery label was required on the e-cigarette product and included a written description of the delivery label requirement. The purpose of delivery labels is to distinguish the contents of the package (e.g., "contains a vapor product") or provide notice of the illegality of sales to minors (e.g., "prohibition on shipping to individuals under 21"). In some states, delivery packaging labels are mandatory in addition to the product packaging warning required by the Food and Drug Administration[25] that details the addictive nature of nicotine, or state warnings listing the potentially negative health risks or harmful ingredients in e-cigarettes, such as toxic metals (e.g., NY Pub Health L §1701).

Permit or Registration Requirement

We identified states that required distinct permits or registrations of e-cigarette sales delivery or remote sales vendors. This is different from, yet could be in addition to, general tobacco retail licensing, as relatively few states require permits or registrations for delivery and remote sales, compared with the many states requiring general tobacco retail licensing.[26]

Fines and Penalties for Violations

Coding included fines and penalties for violations of delivery sales laws. Fines involved monetary amounts according to a set amount, limit, or cost equivalence with retail sales value. Penalties involved license suspension for a fixed period or number of days imprisoned. All fines and penalties apply to sellers or distributors who violated provisions in state delivery sales laws rather than to buyers.

RESULTS

In total, 34 states had e-cigarette delivery sales laws, and the delivery terminology used in these laws is shown in Table A (available as a supplement to the online version of this article at http://www.ajph.org). The most common words used were "delivery," "Internet," and "mail." Of states with coded laws, 29 used "delivery," and the majority explicitly mentioned "Internet," including identifying the terms "electronic network," "computer network," and "online." States also used varying terminology regarding the method of purchase.

Age Verification Requirements

Table 1 shows the heterogeneity in states' age verification requirements at purchase and delivery, with 27 states having at least 1 form of requirement. Regarding age verification at purchase, many states required verification via a database; other means of verification included specific payment types, certification, and proof of government identification. Certain states stipulated age verification upon delivery, with 15 requiring the signature of an adult and 7 needing government identification for the release of the product at delivery. Of the 27 states having requirements, 4 did not explicitly require any form of age verification for purchase, and 11 had no requirements for any age verification upon delivery.

Packaging Label Requirements

Several states required a packaging label for e-cigarette delivery sales (Table 2), with some imposing more stringent labeling requirements. For example, a few statutes specified that the label must display that a "vapor product" is contained inside. Examples of required packaging wording included "electronic nicotine delivery system" (Connecticut), "electronic smoking device" (Idaho), "tobacco substitute" (Delaware), "e-cigarette" (Illinois), and "e-liquids" (Indiana). Certain states specifically required that packaging display a statement that the law prohibited shipping to individuals aged younger than 21 years; in 4 other states, packaging had to display that proof of age was required for delivery.

Permit or Registration Requirements

Table 3 shows states with e-cigarette delivery sales permit or registration requirements, with 7 applying to persons who may engage in the delivery sales of e-cigarettes and 1 statute applying exclusively to out-of-state sellers. Sources for obtaining permits and registrations, such as through alcohol or tobacco control boards, the comptroller, and the Department of Revenue or Finance, also differed by state.

Fines and Penalties for Violations

Table 4 shows the fines and penalties for violations of e-cigarette delivery sales laws. There were considerable

TABLE 1— Age Verification Requirements for E-Cigarette Delivery Sales: United States, 2022

Laws	Effective Dates	Database Purchase	Payment Purchase	Certify Purchase	Gov ID Purchase	Sign Delivery	Gov ID Delivery
Ala Code §13A-12-3.8	August 1, 2019	X	X				
Cal Bus & Prof Code §22963	June 9, 2016	X	X	X	X	X	
Colo Rev Stat §44-7-104.7	July 14, 2020						X
Conn Gen Stat §21a-418	October 1, 2019					X	X
Del Code Ann tit 30 §§5363, 5365	July 16, 2019		X	X	X	X	X
Fla Stat §569.45	October 1, 2021	X	X	X	X	X	X
Ga Code Ann §48-11-4.2	January 1, 2021					X	X
Haw Rev Stat §245-17	July 1, 2018	X		X	X	X	
Idaho Code §39-5715	July 1, 2020	X	X	X			
720 Ill Comp Stats 678/5, 7	January 1, 2022	X	X	X	X	X	X
Ind Code §§7.1-7-6-6, 5.5-3	April 27, 2017	X	X		X		
Iowa Code §453A.47B	July 1, 2017	X			X	X	
940 Mass Code Regs 21.04	September 25, 2015	X				X	
Mich Comp Laws §722.641	September 2, 2019	X					
Miss Code Ann §97-32-51	July 1, 2013	X					
Nev Rev Stat §202.24935	May 27, 2021	X					
NM Stat Ann §61-37-14	January 1, 2021	X					
NC Gen Stat §14-313	August 1, 2013	X					
ND Cent Code §51-32-01	August 1, 2015	X	X	X	X	X	X
Or Rev Stat Ann §323.709	January 1, 2022	X	X	X			
11 RI Gen Laws §11-9-13.11	July 7, 2021			X	X	X	
SC Code Ann §16-17-500	June 7, 2013	X			X	X	
Tenn Code Ann §39-17-1504	July 1, 2015			X			
Tex Health & Safety Code Ann §161.453	October 1, 2015	X	X	X	X	X	
Va Code Ann §18.2-371.2	July 1, 2014	X				X	
Wash Rev Code §70.345.090	June 28, 2016	X	X	X			
Wyo Stat Ann §14-3-309	July 1, 2020	X				X	

Note. "Database Purchase" refers to states requiring age verification for purchase by comparing a customer's provided identity and age with information with public records, a third-party database, or aggregate databases. "Payment Purchase" refers to states requiring payment for purchase through a credit or debit card or a check written in the purchaser's name. "Certify Purchase" refers to states requiring a form of certification for purchase in which the potential purchaser attests that they are of the legal age to make the purchase. "Gov ID Purchase" means that a valid form of government identification was required for delivery purchase and "Gov ID Delivery" means the same requirement, but for the release of the product at delivery. "Sign Delivery" refers to states requiring a signature either by an adult of legal e-cigarette purchasing age or by the specific purchaser of the e-cigarette product for release of the product at delivery.

differences among states having e-cigarette delivery sales laws on how they addressed fines and penalties, and some states also had nonmonetary penalties. No explicit penalties or fines for e-cigarette delivery sales were identified for 5 states. Fines ranged from $10 for a first-time violation by a minor to several thousand dollars for a knowing violation by an adult. Penalties also varied, from a 30-day suspension of authorization to deliver vapor products to imprisonment up to 5 years.

DISCUSSION

Previous studies have addressed diverse e-cigarette regulations in the United States, including tobacco retail licensing laws,[26] aerosol-free indoor laws,[27] e-cigarette taxes,[28] tobacco products definitions,[29] e-cigarette youth access,[22] child-resistant packaging,[30] and others.[23] To our knowledge, no research has comprehensively reviewed e-cigarette delivery sales laws across the United States. Our study fills this gap in

TABLE 2— Packaging Label Requirements for E-Cigarette Delivery Sales: United States, 2022

Laws	Effective Dates	Packaging Label Requirement
Cal Bus & Prof Code §22963	January 1, 2020	"Contains tobacco products: Signature of person 21 years of age or older required for delivery."
Conn Gen Stat §21a-418	October 1, 2019	"Contains an electronic nicotine delivery system or vapor product—signature of a person 21 or older required for delivery."
Del Code Ann tit 30 §5365	July 16, 2019	"Any Tobacco Product or Tobacco Substitute: Delaware Law Prohibits Shipping to Individuals Under 21, and Requires the Payment of all Applicable Taxes."
Fla Stat §569.45	October 1, 2021	"Nicotine Products: Florida law prohibits shipping to individuals under 21 years of age."
Idaho Code §39-5717	July 1, 2020	"Tobacco products or electronic smoking devices: Idaho law prohibits shipping to individuals under the age of twenty-one (21) years and requires the payment of taxes pursuant to chapter 25, title 63, Idaho Code. Persons violating this law may be civilly and criminally liable."
720 Ill Comp Stats 678/7	January 1, 2022	"Cigarettes or electronic cigarettes: Illinois Law Prohibits Shipping to Individuals Under 21 and Requires the Payment of All Applicable Taxes."
Ind Code §7.1-7-5.5-5	April 27, 2017	"E-liquids: Indiana law prohibits the sale of this product to a person who is less than 21 years of age."
Nev Rev Stat §202.24935	May 27, 2021	Packaging or wrapping of items when they are shipped to be clearly marked with the words "tobacco products," "vapor products" or "nicotine products," as applicable.
NY Pub Health Law §1399-LL	July 1, 2020	Any shipping of vapor products other than in manufacturer's original container or wrapping, the container or wrapping must be plainly and visibly marked with the words "vapor products."
Or Rev Stat Ann. §323.715	January 1, 2022	Notice including prominent and clearly legible statement that: 1) "tobacco sales to persons under [the legal minimum purchase age] 21 years of age are illegal;" 2) "sales of tobacco are restricted to those individuals who provide verifiable proof of age in accordance with ORS 323.709;" and 3) "sales of other tobacco products are subject to tax under ORS 323.500 to 323.645, and an explanation of how the applicable tax has been paid or is to be paid."
Tex Health & Safety Code Ann §161.454	October 1, 2015	Delivery sale must include prominent and clearly legible statement that: "(1) e-cigarette sales to individuals younger than the age prescribed by Section 161.082 are illegal under state law; and (2) e-cigarette sales are restricted to individuals who provide verifiable proof of age in accordance with Section 161.453."
Wash Rev Code §70.345.090	June 28, 2016	A delivery sale licensee must include on shipping documents a clear and conspicuous statement which includes, at a minimum, that the package contains vapor products, Washington law prohibits sales to those under the minimum age established by the chapter, and violations may result in sanctions to both the licensee and the purchaser.

the extant literature. Moreover, this study contributes to a growing body of literature focused on e-cigarette laws by cataloging the US e-cigarette delivery sales laws, which scholars and policymakers will find useful for discerning these policies' impact and informing effective future regulatory decisions.

Our findings reveal extensive variability in e-cigarette delivery sales laws among states. We found considerable heterogeneity in states' e-cigarette delivery sales laws, particularly regarding the scope and dimensions of the laws. Some states specified a comprehensive list of restricted purchase methods (e.g., Internet, mail, phone, voice, and fax), whereas others were narrower in scope or had no relevant laws. Likewise, certain states required an array of age verification procedures, whereas others only required 1 form of age verification, either at the point of purchase or at delivery. Among the few states mandating packaging labels on e-cigarette delivery, some mandated language regarding contents (e.g., e-liquid, tobacco product, vapor product, electronic nicotine delivery system), age restrictions (e.g., underage prohibitions vs signature requirements), or tax payments. Similarly, there was inconsistency in the type of permits or registration needed for e-cigarette delivery. States varied widely in fines and severity of penalties for violations of e-cigarette delivery laws, ranging from several hundred dollars in fines to treatment of violations as small misdemeanors or felonies.

Although most state laws that we examined extend beyond the federal requirements, mapping this range of regulatory approaches reveals potential loopholes that may diminish these laws' effectiveness. First, major mail carriers (e.g., United Parcel Service, DHL, FedEx) in 2021 voluntarily stopped deliveries of all e-cigarette products in

TABLE 3— Permit or Registration Requirements for E-Cigarette Delivery Sales: United States, 2022

Laws	Effective Dates	Permit and Registration Requirements
Ala Code §13A-12–3.8	August 1, 2019	"No person may conduct a delivery sale of electronic nicotine delivery systems or alternative nicotine products unless the seller has obtained a valid permit to conduct delivery sales of electronic nicotine delivery systems or alternative nicotine products issued by the board pursuant to Section 28-11-4."
Ark Code Ann §26–57-214	July 22, 2015	"A person shall not deal with, deliver or cause to be delivered to a retailer or consumer, or otherwise do business in tobacco products, vapor products, alternative nicotine products, or e-liquid products in this state without first registering with the Director of Arkansas Tobacco Control and obtaining a permit for that purpose."
Del Code Ann tit 30 §5366	July 16, 2019	"Prior to making delivery sales or mailing, shipping or otherwise delivering any tobacco product, as defined under § 5301 of this title, in connection with any such sales, every person shall file with the Department a statement setting forth such person's name, trade name and the address of such person's principal place of business and any other place of business."
Minn Stat §297F.031	January 1, 2022	"Prior to making delivery sales, an out-of-state retailer must file with the Department of Revenue a statement setting forth the out-of-state retailer's name, trade name, address, principal place of business, and any other place of business."
Or Rev Stat Ann §323.712	January 1, 2022	"A person may not engage in delivery sales of tobacco in this state without first obtaining the applicable distributor's license under ORS 323.105 or 323.530 and any applicable retailer's license required by a jurisdiction into which a delivery sale of tobacco is made."
Tex Health & Safety Code Ann §161.456	October 1, 2015	"A person may not make a delivery sale or ship cigarettes or e-cigarettes in connection with a delivery sale unless the person first files with the comptroller a statement that includes: (1) the person's name and trade name; and (2) the address of the person's principal place of business and any other place of business, and the person's telephone number and e-mail address."
Wash Rev Code §70.345.090	June 28, 2016	"No person may conduct a delivery sale or otherwise ship or transport, or cause to be shipped or transported, any vapor product ordered or purchased by mail or through the internet to any person unless such seller has a valid delivery sale license as required under this chapter."

light of the federal Preventing Online Sales of E-Cigarettes to Children Act. However, many e-cigarette businesses continue to make arrangements with private transportation and logistics companies,[20] or otherwise find and utilize various legal ambiguities to sustain delivery sales.[31] For example, 1 Internet-based brand uses its employees or independent contractors to drive household items directly to consumers,[31] offering over a hundred vape and vaping products for delivery on demand.[32] This arrangement raises concern over the proverbial fox guarding the henhouse. Second, as with any law, ambiguities can be exploited if legal terminology is not explicit.[29] For instance, a state that restricts delivery sales through Internet purchases but does not include purchases made through phone communication will be vulnerable to unregulated youth access. Likewise, a state that requires age verification for purchase but not delivery is susceptible to e-cigarettes potentially getting into the hands of minors. Third, compliance and enforcement present real-world implementation challenges. Significant resources would be needed to extensively surveil online e-cigarette businesses for compliance. Additionally, the vast number of e-cigarette brands, products, and accessories[33,34] makes online enforcement difficult.

Limitations

Several limitations to this study are noteworthy. E-cigarette delivery sales laws were not always easy to locate. For instance, relevant statutes were located under diverse titles, including "health and safety," "criminal codes," or "taxation," or mentioned as an isolated subsection within a broader chapter concerned with safeguarding public morals or protecting minors from tobacco. In some states, however, e-cigarette delivery statutes are discrete sections within chapters titled "Delivery Sales," "Tobacco Delivery Sales," or other straightforward labels. Because of the inconsistency in how states framed the law, our data collection may have missed some relevant laws. Furthermore, the e-cigarette regulatory environment evolves rapidly, and the review provided here represents a snapshot of current laws. Lastly, this study focused solely on cataloging e-cigarette delivery laws; it did not seek to document the extent or effectiveness of state enforcement of these laws. Future studies could examine how these laws are enforced, including capturing

TABLE 4— Fines and Penalties for Violations for E-Cigarette Delivery Sales: United States, 2022

Laws	Effective Dates	Fines	Penalties
Ala Code §13A-12-3.8	August 1, 2019	First: $100–500 Subsequent: $500–1 500	
Ark Code Ann §§5-4-201, 5-4-401	July 22, 2015	Not more than $2 500	Not to exceed 1 y in prison
Cal Bus & Prof Code §22963	June 9, 2016	First violation: $1 000–2 000 Second: $2 500–3 500 Third (within 5 y): $4 000–5 000 Fourth (within 5 y): $5 500–6 500 Fifth (within 5 y): $10 000	
Colo Rev Stat §44-7-106	July 14, 2020	First: $1 000 Second (within 24 mo): $2 000 Third (within 24 mo): $3 000	If more than 3 violations within 24 mo, order given prohibiting retailer from selling tobacco or nicotine products. Retailer then ineligible to apply for state licensure for 3 y
Del Code Ann tit 30 §5368	July 16, 2019	First: $1 000 or 5 times the retail value of product (whichever is greater) Second or subsequent: $5 000 or 5 times the retail value (whichever is greater) Knowingly violates provisions: A) $10 000 or 5 times the retail value	Knowingly violates provisions: B) imprisoned less than 5 y, or C) both A and B
Fla Stat §§775.082, 775.083	October 1, 2021	Knowing violation: misdemeanor second degree: $500	Knowing violation: misdemeanor second degree: less than 60 d prison
Ga Code Ann §48-11-4.2	January 1, 2021	Up to $500 for each	Up to 30-d suspension for each violation
Haw Rev Sta. §245-17	July 1, 2018	First (≥ 21 y): $500 Subsequent (≥ 21 y): $500–2000 First (< 21 y): $10 Subsequent (< 21 y): $50	Subsequent (< 21 y): 48–72 h community service
720 Ill Comp. Stats 678/10	January 1, 2022	Not more than $5 000	First: class A misdemeanor Subsequent: class 4 felony
Ind Code §35-50-3-4	April 27, 2017	Not more than $500	Class C misdemeanor up to 60 d imprisoned
Iowa Code §453A.50	July 1, 2017	First: $200 Second (within 3 y): $500 Third or subsequent (within 3 y): $1 000	
Me Rev Stat An. tit 22 §1555-F	November 1, 2017	Not less than $1 000 and not more than $5 000 for each violation	
Mich Comp Laws §722.641	September 2, 2019	First: not more than $100 Second: not more than $500 Third or subsequent: not more than $2 500	
Miss Code Ann §97-32-51	July 1, 2013	First: $250 Second: $500 Third or subsequent: $1 000	
Nev Rev Stat §202.24935	May 27, 2021	Not more than $1 000 per violation	Suspension or revocation of license by Department of Taxation if licensed
NY Pub Health Law §1399-LL	July 1, 2020	Not more than $5 000 per violation and $100 per each vapor product shipped	First: class A misdemeanor Second or subsequent: class E felony
NC Gen Stat §105-113.4F	October 1, 2019	First: $1 000 Subsequent: not to exceed $5 000	
ND Cent Code § 51-32-07	August 1, 2015	First: not more than $1 000 Second or subsequent: $1 000-$5 000	Knowingly violates: class C felony
Or Rev Stat Ann §323.727	January 1, 2022	First: $1 000 or 5 times the retail value of product (whichever is greater) Second or subsequent: $5 000 or 5 times the retail value of product (whichever is greater) Knowing violation: A) $10 000 or 5 times the retail value of product (whichever is greater)	Knowing violation: B) imprisoned less than 5 y

Continued

TABLE 4— Continued

Laws	Effective Dates	Fines	Penalties
11 RI Gen Laws §11-9-13.11	July 7, 2021	Minimum $1 000 for each delivery to anyone younger than 21 y	
SC Code Ann §16-17-500	June 7, 2013	First: $200–300 Second and subsequent: A) $400–500	Second and subsequent: B) 30 d imprisoned
SD Cod Laws §10-50-101	July 1, 2019	First: $1 000 or 5 times the retail value of product Subsequent: $5 000 or 5 times the retail value of product	
Tenn Code Ann § 39-17-1509	July 1, 2015	First: warning letter Second: not more than $500 (within 5 y) Third: not more than $1 000 (within 5 y) Fourth: not more than $1 500 (within 5 y)	
Tex Pen Codes §§12.22, 12.23	October 1, 2015	First: not to exceed $500 Subsequent: A) not to exceed $2 000	First: class C misdemeanor Subsequent: B) 180 d in jail or C) both A and B
Utah Code Ann §59-14-808	July 1, 2020	Not to exceed $5 000 for each knowing violation	
Vt Stat Ann tit 7 §1010	July 1, 2019	Not to exceed $5 000 for each	
Va Code Ann §18.2-371.2	July 1, 2014	First: not to exceed $100 Second: not to exceed $200 Third or subsequent: $500	
Wash Rev Code §70.345.090	June 28, 2016	Up to $5 000 for each	Class C felony
Wyo Stat Ann §14-3-302	July 1, 2020	First (within 24 mo): $250 Second (within 24 mo): $500 Third or subsequent (within 24 mo): $750	Injunction prohibiting selling for up to 180 d

variation in communities. Notwithstanding these limitations, this study offers a comprehensive mapping of state e-cigarette delivery sales laws.

Public Health Implications

Underage e-cigarette use is an ongoing public health concern. In September 2022, a popular e-cigarette brand settled out of court and agreed to pay over $400 million to 34 states and territories investigating its marketing efforts, including social media campaigns, for specifically targeting young people.[35] Many tobacco product access laws have been in effect for nearly a decade in some states, addressing prohibitions on flavoring and on sales and marketing to minors, mandates of health warnings and child-proof packaging, vape-free policies, and venue and location regulations.[23] Without proper regulatory safeguards involving e-cigarette prevention and control, such underage access continues to threaten future generations' public health. Furthermore, if retail store access laws are more restrictive than e-commerce laws, motivated youths will be incentivized to exploit the lax nonretail access.

Even though there is no one-size-fits-all approach, stringent policy regimes with fewer loopholes will likely be more effective at enforcing youth access prevention. For example, states could use more precise terminology to prohibit all forms of delivery sales. Similarly, many states could include more age verification requirements to cover both the point of purchase and delivery of e-cigarette products. Permit and registration requirements would allow states to monitor delivery efficiently and guard against unscrupulous activities. States could more explicitly convey that e-cigarette delivery and sale to underage persons is a severe violation with appropriate consequences, and a summary of penalties on the shipment's packaging could be an effective education tool. Finally, fines and penalties could be enhanced to prevent the selling of products to underage consumers. AJPH

ABOUT THE AUTHORS

Sunday Azagba, Todd Ebling, and Olayemi Timothy Adekeye are with the Ross and Carol Nese College of Nursing, Pennsylvania State University, University Park. Mark Hall is with the Department of Social Science and Health Policy, Wake Forest School of Medicine, Winston-Salem, NC. Jessica King Jensen is with the Department of Health and Kinesiology, University of Utah, Salt Lake City.

CORRESPONDENCE

Correspondence should be sent to Sunday Azagba, College of Nursing, University Park, PA 16802 (e-mail: spa5695@psu.edu). Reprints can be ordered at http://www.ajph.org by clicking the "Reprints" link.

PUBLICATION INFORMATION

Full Citation: Azagba S, Ebling T, Adekeye OT, Hall M, Jensen JK. Loopholes for underage access in e-cigarette delivery sales laws, United States, 2022. *Am J Public Health*. 2023;113(5):568–576.

Acceptance Date: January 3, 2023.

DOI: https://doi.org/10.2105/AJPH.2023.307228

CONTRIBUTORS

S. Azagba obtained funding and designed and conceptualized the study. T. Ebling was involved in the conceptualization. T. Ebling, O. T Adekeye, and S. Azagba coded the laws. S. Azagba, T. Ebling, M. Hall, and J. K. Jensen contributed to the article drafting and interpretation of findings. All authors thoroughly reviewed the article and approved this version.

ACKNOWLEDGMENTS

Publication of this research was supported by funding from the National Cancer Institute (R01CA249052) to S. Azagba.

Note. The sponsors had no role in the design and conduct of the study; in the collection, management, analysis, and interpretation of the data; in the preparation, review, or approval of the article; or the decision to submit the manuscript for publication.

CONFLICTS OF INTEREST

The authors have no conflicts of interest to disclose.

HUMAN PARTICIPANT PROTECTION

No protocol approval was necessary because data were obtained from secondary sources.

REFERENCES

1. Cohen JE, Sarabia V, Ashley MJ. Tobacco commerce on the internet: a threat to comprehensive tobacco control. *Tob Control*. 2001;10(4):364–367. https://doi.org/10.1136/tc.10.4.364
2. Ribisl KM. The potential of the internet as a medium to encourage and discourage youth tobacco use. *Tob Control*. 2003;12(suppl 1):i48–i59. https://doi.org/10.1136/tc.12.suppl_1.i48
3. Jensen JA, Hickman NJ III, Landrine H, Klonoff EA. Availability of tobacco to youth via the internet. *JAMA*. 2004;291(15):1837. https://doi.org/10.1001/jama.291.15.1837
4. Chriqui J, Ribisl K, Wallace R, Williams R, O'Connor J, el Arculli R. A comprehensive review of state laws governing Internet and other delivery sales of cigarettes in the United States. *Nicotine Tob Res*. 2008;10(2):253–265. https://doi.org/10.1080/14622200701838232
5. Gentzke AS. Vital signs: tobacco product use among middle and high school students—United States, 2011–2018. *MMWR Morb Mortal Wkly Rep*. 2019;68(6):157–164. https://doi.org/10.15585/mmwr.mm6806e1
6. Cooper M. Notes from the field: e-cigarette use among middle and high school students—United States, 2022. *MMWR Morb Mortal Wkly Rep*. 2022;71(40):1283–1285. https://doi.org/10.15585/mmwr.mm7140a3
7. *E-Cigarette Use Among Youth and Young Adults: A Report of the Surgeon General—Executive Summary*. Atlanta, GA: US Dept of Health and Human Services, Centers for Disease Control and Prevention; 2016.
8. Chun LF, Moazed F, Calfee CS, Matthay MA, Gotts JE. Pulmonary toxicity of e-cigarettes. *Am J Physiol Lung Cell Mol Physiol*. 2017;313(2):L193–L206. https://doi.org/10.1152/ajplung.00071.2017
9. Cameron JM, Howell DN, White JR, Andrenyak DM, Layton ME, Roll JM. Variable and potentially fatal amounts of nicotine in e-cigarette nicotine solutions. *Tob Control*. 2014;23(1):77–78. https://doi.org/10.1136/tobaccocontrol-2012-050604
10. Goniewicz ML, Hajek P, McRobbie H. Nicotine content of electronic cigarettes, its release in vapour and its consistency across batches: regulatory implications. *Addiction*. 2014;109(3):500–507. https://doi.org/10.1111/add.12410
11. Mackey TK, Miner A, Cuomo RE. Exploring the e-cigarette e-commerce marketplace: identifying internet e-cigarette marketing characteristics and regulatory gaps. *Drug Alcohol Depend*. 2015;156:97–103. https://doi.org/10.1016/j.drugalcdep.2015.08.032
12. Zhu SH, Sun JY, Bonnevie E, et al. Four hundred and sixty brands of e-cigarettes and counting: implications for product regulation. *Tob Control*. 2014;23(suppl 3):iii3–iii9. https://doi.org/10.1136/tobaccocontrol-2014-051670
13. Williams RS, Derrick J, Ribisl KM. Electronic cigarette sales to minors via the internet. *JAMA Pediatr*. 2015;169(3):e1563. https://doi.org/10.1001/jamapediatrics.2015.63
14. Pepper JK, Coats EM, Nonnemaker JM, Loomis BR. How do adolescents get their e-cigarettes and other electronic vaping devices? *Am J Health Promot*. 2019;33(3):420–429. https://doi.org/10.1177/0890117118790366
15. King JL, Merten JW, Nicksic NE. Who purchases tobacco online? Findings from waves 1 and 4 of the Population Assessment of Tobacco and Health Study. *Tob Regul Sci*. 2021;7(3):155–169. https://doi.org/10.18001/TRS.7.3.1
16. Ramamurthi D, Chau C, Jackler RK. Exploitation of the COVID-19 pandemic by e-cigarette marketers. *Tob Control*. 2021;30(e1):e56–e59. https://doi.org/10.1136/tobaccocontrol-2020-055855
17. Pokhrel P, Fagan P, Herzog TA, et al. Social media e-cigarette exposure and e-cigarette expectancies and use among young adults. *Addict Behav*. 2018;78:51–58. https://doi.org/10.1016/j.addbeh.2017.10.017
18. Public Health Law Center. Return to sender: e-cigarette delivery sales in 2021. 2021. Available at: https://www.publichealthlawcenter.org/sites/default/files/resources/Return-To-Sender-PACT-Act.pdf. Accessed September 22, 2022.
19. Freight Right. UPS, DHL, and FedEx join USPS in vape mail ban. 2021. Available at: https://www.freightright.com/news/vape-mail-ban. Accessed September 26, 2022.
20. National Law Review. Congress amends the PACT Act to apply to all vaping products, placing huge burden on small manufacturers as third-party common carriers refuse to ship products. Available at: https://www.natlawreview.com/article/congress-amends-pact-act-to-apply-to-all-vaping-products-placing-huge-burden-small. Accessed August 16, 2022.
21. Williams RS, Derrick J, Phillips KJ. Cigarette sales to minors via the internet: how the story has changed in the wake of federal regulation. *Tob Control*. 2017;26(4):415–420. https://doi.org/10.1136/tobaccocontrol-2015-052844
22. Gourdet CK, Chriqui JF, Chaloupka FJ. A baseline understanding of state laws governing e-cigarettes. *Tob Control*. 2014;23(suppl 3):iii37–iii40. https://doi.org/10.1136/tobaccocontrol-2013-051459
23. Dobbs PD, Hammig B, Sudduth A. 2015 legislative update of e-cigarette youth access and exposure laws. *Prev Med*. 2016;88:90–94. https://doi.org/10.1016/j.ypmed.2016.03.010
24. Public Health Law Center. US e-cigarette regulation: a 50-state review. Available at: https://www.publichealthlawcenter.org/sites/default/files/inline-files/ECigarette-Legal-Landscape-June15-2022.pdf. Accessed September 21, 2022.
25. King JL, Lazard A, Reboussin BA, et al. Optimizing warnings on e-cigarette advertisements. *Nicotine Tob Res*. 2020;22(5):630–637. https://doi.org/10.1093/ntr/ntz091
26. Patel M, Donovan EM, Perks SN, et al. E-cigarette tobacco retail licensing laws: variance across US states as of January 1, 2020. *Am J Public Health*. 2020;110(9):1380–1385. https://doi.org/10.2105/AJPH.2020.305771
27. Lee B, Lin HC, Seo DC. Inclusion of electronic nicotine delivery systems in indoor smoke-free air policies and associated vaping behavior. *Addict Behav*. 2019;98:106061. https://doi.org/10.1016/j.addbeh.2019.106061
28. Cotti C, Nesson E, Pesko MF, Phillips S, Tefft N. Standardising the measurement of e-cigarette taxes in the USA, 2010–2020. *Tob Control*. 2021; Epub ahead of print. https://doi.org/10.1136/tobaccocontrol-2021-056865
29. Lempert LK, Grana R, Glantz SA. The importance of product definitions in US e-cigarette laws and regulations. *Tob Control*. 2016;25(e1):e44–e51. https://doi.org/10.1136/tobaccocontrol-2014-051913
30. Govindarajan P, Spiller HA, Casavant MJ, Chounthirath T, Smith GA. E-cigarette and liquid nicotine exposures among young children. *Pediatrics*. 2018;141(5):e20173361. https://doi.org/10.1542/peds.2017-3361
31. Public Health Law Center. Online sales of e-cigarettes & other tobacco products. 2022. Available at: https://www.publichealthlawcenter.org/sites/default/files/resources/Online-Sales-E-Cigarettes-Other-Tobacco-Products.pdf. Accessed August 17, 2022.
32. Gopuff Web site. Available at: https://www.gopuff.com/search?q=vape. Accessed September 26, 2022.
33. Ali FRM, Diaz MC, Vallone D, et al. E-cigarette unit sales, by product and flavor type—United States, 2014–2020. *MMWR Morb Mortal Wkly Rep*. 2020;69(37):1313–1318. https://doi.org/10.15585/mmwr.mm6937e2
34. Krishnan-Sarin S, Jackson A, Morean M, et al. E-cigarette devices used by high-school youth. *Drug Alcohol Depend*. 2019;194:395–400. https://doi.org/10.1016/j.drugalcdep.2018.10.022
35. Christensen J. Juul to pay $438.5 million in settlement with dozens of states over marketing to underage people. CNN. September 6, 2022. Available at: https://www.cnn.com/2022/09/06/health/juul-settlement-marketing/index.html. Accessed September 20, 2022.

Ethics Principles for Artificial Intelligence–Based Telemedicine for Public Health

Simona Tiribelli, PhD, Annabelle Monnot, MSc, Syed F. H. Shah, BA, MB BChir, Anmol Arora, MB BChir, Ping J. Toong, and Sokanha Kong, MPhil

See also Kraft, p. 470.

The use of artificial intelligence (AI) in the field of telemedicine has grown exponentially over the past decade, along with the adoption of AI-based telemedicine to support public health systems.

Although AI-based telemedicine can open up novel opportunities for the delivery of clinical health and care and become a strong aid to public health systems worldwide, it also comes with ethical risks that should be detected, prevented, or mitigated for the responsible use of AI-based telemedicine in and for public health. However, despite the current proliferation of AI ethics frameworks, thus far, none have been developed for the design of AI-based telemedicine, especially for the adoption of AI-based telemedicine in and for public health.

We aimed to fill this gap by mapping the most relevant AI ethics principles for AI-based telemedicine for public health and by showing the need to revise them via major ethical themes emerging from bioethics, medical ethics, and public health ethics toward the definition of a unified set of 6 AI ethics principles for the implementation of AI-based telemedicine. (*Am J Public Health*. 2023;113(5):577–584. https://doi.org/10.2105/AJPH.2023.307225)

AJPH May 2023, Vol 113, No. 5

The increasingly widespread availability of digital devices has facilitated the growth of telehealth and telemedicine over the past few decades, which is broadly described by the US Centers for Disease Control and Prevention (CDC) as "the use of electronic information and telecommunication technologies to support and promote long-distance clinical health care, patient and professional health-related education, public health, and health administration."[1] In particular, the development and adoption of telehealth and telemedicine were exponentially accelerated by the COVID-19 pandemic, with the CDC reporting a 50% and 154% increase in teleconsultations in January 2020 and March 2020, respectively, compared with the same periods in 2019. This was arguably the most substantial and large-scale proof of the value of telehealth and telemedicine in ensuring prevention and other health services for diverse communities worldwide—especially in times of global health crises[2]—and proof of their potential benefit for global public health.[3]

In parallel, the field of artificial intelligence (AI) and its applications to the health and medical domains have been expanding rapidly because of improvements in the hardware capabilities of modern computer systems, the pervasive applications of information and communication technologies (ICTs), and the consequent digitalization of health data and records. "AI" is an umbrella term conventionally used to refer to the ability of computer systems to perform tasks that are usually thought to require human skills, including reasoning and self-correction.[4]

AI and, specifically, probabilistic machine learning (ML) algorithms—models that learn novel correlations and patterns from the collection and mining of huge streams of data to execute tasks, decisions, and predictions—are now being developed in nearly all domains of public health and medical practice.[4] These include, but are not limited to, diagnostic support, remote monitoring, prediction and detection, robot-assisted treatments, and biomedical research.[5] In all these diverse applications, ML presents a huge opportunity to supplement or enhance remote health services via telehealth devices and telemedicine solutions, which we particularly address in this article. Indeed, although telemedicine and telehealth overlap greatly and many prefer to use such terms interchangeably, there is an often undervalued but key distinction between the 2 domains, which experts in the field and public health bodies such as the World Health Organization (WHO) also advocate.[6,7]

TAXONOMY

"Telehealth" is used in reference to the broad delivery of health care services via ICTs, including devices for health care self-management (i.e., with clinicians or health care providers [HCPs] out of the loop), whereas "telemedicine" is a subset of telehealth and refers to more clinical-oriented health care delivery via ICTs that include the intervention of a clinician in a synchronous way (e.g., teleconsultation) or in an asynchronous modality (e.g., store and forward telemedicine).[7] Indeed, "telehealth" also includes nonclinical services, such as virtual education, HCP and clinician training, and health self-management (e.g., fitness trackers). "Telemedicine" refers more specifically to ICTs used for delivering clinical-oriented services for medicine and health care at a distance, and it always requires interfacing between clinicians and patients (or patients' data) for clinical decision-making, which is based on evidence resulting from information obtained via patients' data or clinician–patient conversation (i.e., teleconsultation).[6,7]

ARTIFICIAL INTELLIGENCE, TELEMEDICINE, AND PUBLIC HEALTH

In the field of telemedicine, AI opens up great opportunities that can go beyond those of traditional (i.e., non-AI) telemedicine,[8] such as reducing public health facilities' clinical overload and breaking down barriers that prevent readily accessing public health facilities from a socioeconomic (e.g., in developing areas of the world), health (e.g., patients with severe or chronic illnesses), or geographical (e.g., medical deserts) standpoint.[9]

Indeed, the large amount of health data on individuals (i.e., patient-level data) and populations (i.e., aggregated data) that can be collected by remote monitoring AI-based devices, as well as during AI-empowered teleconsultations, can be used to discover valuable knowledge (e.g., correlations and patterns) that is difficult or expensive to obtain by human manual programming.[10] This knowledge can be harnessed to build preventive and predictive models for personalized health and health care, at both the individual level (i.e., precision clinical treatments)[11] and the population level, enabling public health interventions targeting only certain segments of populations or societies (i.e., precision public health).[12] From this perspective, AI-based telemedicine might become very useful in clinical care and public health systems worldwide.[13,14]

THE ROLE OF ARTIFICIAL INTELLIGENCE ETHICS

However, alongside the rapid growth of interest in the use of AI and ML specifically for telemedicine, there is an emerging awareness that they come with ethical risks. Such risks range from exacerbating discrimination and health inequity because of flawed or biased data sets used to feed and train ML models[15,16] to infringing on patients' autonomy as a result of the misuse of people's health data for third-party economic interests.[17] Although the early literature has suggested specific ethical risks raised by the use of AI broadly and in health care specifically, there is a paucity of ethical research discussing the risks in the specific context of AI-based telemedicine used in and for public health. If such risks remain unaddressed, the huge potential for AI-based telemedicine systems to truly become forces for public health will be deeply compromised. In this regard, public health organizations and practitioners, as well as scholars from a wide range of fields affected by AI, agree on the value of ethics or AI ethics principles on which policy and legal regulation can rely to help detect, prevent, and mitigate AI's risks to people and responsibly orient the design and adoption of AI-based systems for social good and health.[17–20] However, thus far, no ethical framework has been developed for AI-based telemedicine or for AI-based telemedicine for public health.

We sought to fill this gap by highlighting the first, to our knowledge, unified framework of ethical principles to consider, revise or expand, and operationalize to responsibly develop and deploy AI-based telemedicine for public health. To this aim, we first discuss the synergy between AI and telemedicine.

Second, we show the results of mapping and analyzing the main ethical frameworks and related principles (or themes) underpinning the diverse fields brought into play by AI-based telemedicine for public health. By showing both overlaps and differences between principles, and in particular the different ethical connotations and requirements that ethical principles entail in the diverse fields considered, we identify and describe an overarching set of 6

AJPH May 2023, Vol 113, No. 5

agreed-upon AI ethics principles that emerge as relevant for the design and use of AI-based telemedicine for public health.

Third, we selectively use some of the proposed principles to analyze a real-world AI-based telemedicine application and show how such principles allow us to highlight context-sensitive considerations and risks. This analysis also shows that the principles identified for the design and implementation of AI-based telemedicine for public health require further exploration and refinement in a timely way to be truly effective.

ARTIFICIAL INTELLIGENCE IN TELEMEDICINE

The opportunities that AI-based telemedicine systems can offer in terms of processing large amounts of data, improving efficiency, supporting clinical decisions and patients' management, and improving health equity[21] are increasingly acknowledged in the fields of telemedicine and public health.[22] However, because of the rapid advances in AI, only a few comprehensive and up-to-date overviews of AI-empowered telemedicine applications exist in the literature.[10] These applications can be grouped into 3 categories according to their specific clinical-oriented health and health care function.

Remote Diagnosis

Remote diagnosis support tools are increasingly being used to make recommendations for disease screening, diagnosis, treatment, or prevention without requiring as much in-person contact with clinicians or other HCPs as previously. These recommendations are based on large amounts of patient data, ranging from personal or family medical history to imaging that can be acquired remotely. Thus, such tools can advance health equity by promoting access to public health facilities and clinical treatments, especially for those living in underserved communities or affected by severe illness.[23] Patients can use some of these tools directly without the synchronous presence of clinicians or HCPs; for example, they can hold conversations with chatbots that use natural language processing to gain information about their conditions for transmission to HCPs.

An example of such tools in public health include SGDormBot (Bot MD, Singapore), an AI-based telemedicine tool used during the COVID-19 pandemic that used a WhatsApp chatline for real-time symptom-based mass screening of migrant workers' health in Singapore for prompt clinical intervention.[24] For other tools, the end users are clinicians, as in teleophthalmology, wherein clinicians receive patients' data, which was gathered in home environments, and evaluate them as diagnostic support.[25] To support clinicians' diagnoses, other AI-based tools, such as health recommender systems, may be used to generate treatment recommendations according to models built on the data of different interventions for patients with distinct characteristics and their associated outcomes.

Virtual Consultations

The infrastructure underlying telemedicine is becoming increasingly sophisticated, with an increase in teleconsultation platforms and digitalization of medical records. Teleconsultations have been widely perceived to increase patient convenience by reducing travel and wait time. Teleconsultations are increasingly based on AI-powered online platforms with features that aid physicians in their work and improve the experience of virtual medical consultation. One such feature is automated speech recognition and recording based on ML, which can process speech and translate it into clinical documentation. Such platforms, when based on natural language processing, can even extract the sentiment of recorded dialogue, helping with documenting medical notes, patient history, and medical data. Today, such tools often embed facial recognition algorithms for emotion recognition that enable clinicians to test patients' emotional status and their understanding of health issues.

Babylon Health (Babylon Health, London, UK) is a prime example of an AI-based telemedicine tool embedding such features adopted to support the UK National Health Service. Electronic health records also have the potential to be augmented via AI, with ML techniques, such as collaborative filtering, that can detect new trends and predict health outcomes at the individual and collective levels. Finally, algorithms may help optimize triaging of patients to the most relevant HCPs, thereby reducing hospital overload while boosting patients' health and care management.[26]

Remote Monitoring and Management

Remote monitoring and management usually consists of a system that can gather, process, and transmit data between an outpatient and their HCPs.[27] Data acquisition by implanted or worn devices or smartphone apps is paired with ML-powered analytic capabilities that integrate data streams into clinical workflows for HCPs to make proactive adjustments and predictions and give personalized feedback. Remote monitoring systems are especially useful for monitoring conditions such as diabetes, heart failure, and Parkinson's disease and, in postsurgical rehabilitation, for empowering those living in oppressive health conditions.

An example of such a system with relevance to public health is the human activity recognition system, which consists of sensors set up in patients' rooms to allow remote monitoring of residents in assisted living facilities or care homes.[28] The AI-powered sensors can note the different functional states of residents and present recommendations to HCPs to avoid falls and heart attacks and to make adjustments to medication regimes, overcoming sociorelational limits imposed by geographical distance.

KEY ETHICAL PRINCIPLES

Although AI-powered telemedicine applications are varied and have the potential to radically improve health equity, clinical care, and public health systems broadly, they might have ethical risks; therefore, the development and adoption of ethical frameworks is fundamental to detect and tackle such risks. Although more than 84 AI ethics frameworks have been developed worldwide,[29] none have been developed specifically for AI-based telemedicine for public health, despite the increasingly acknowledged importance of the topic both in telemedicine and public health.[19–21,30–33]

To fill this gap, we analyzed different ethical frameworks developed in AI ethics,[17,19,29] bioethics and medical ethics (telehealth and telemedicine included),[33–36] and public health ethics[37,38] and tried to find intersections that might help in the development of a specific ethical framework for AI-based telemedicine for public health. Our analysis showed that all the frameworks rely on the 4 ethical pillars rooted in bioethics: (1) beneficence, (2) nonmaleficence, (3) autonomy, and (4) justice. Our analysis also showed that the main ethical principles and themes discussed in the before-mentioned fields can converge under the macrocategories or high-level principles provided by the WHO in 2021 in its document "Ethics and Governance of Artificial Intelligence for Health."[19]

In Box 1 (see also Table A, available as a supplement to the online version of this article at http://www.ajph.org), we list the WHO's 6 high-level ethical principles and revise them by matching them with the relevant fields in AI-based telemedicine for public health. We also consider what actors are called into action to respect and implement each principle. We provide a brief description of what each principle might prescribe in the context of AI-based telemedicine for public health.

Beneficence and Nonmaleficence

Beneficence and nonmaleficence relate to the doctrines of delivering patient care and aiming to do good and not do harm. Although beneficence is a natural aspect of any proposed medical and public health intervention, nonmaleficence can raise questions in the context of AI-based telemedicine. In fact, some solutions might exhibit a certain degree of maleficence toward vulnerable groups despite being driven by benevolent intentions, for example, when minority groups or those without access to the required technology are excluded from the benefits of digital innovation. To detect potential harms, nonmaleficence ought to be thought of and implemented along with clinical safety, efficacy, and digital inclusion.

Autonomy

Autonomy describes the principle by which individuals should be able to make informed decisions about their own care and requires asking for informed consent and privacy. In this context, AI and public health principles may conflict on the issue of data sharing. AI is a data-driven technology that must be trained on large data sets from diverse populations to work efficiently and avoid biased ML. However, there is often a reluctance to share data because of lack of trust in (health) institutions, especially in certain demographic groups. From a public health perspective, many argue that data sharing for ML training should be made compulsory when these algorithms are to be used at a population level. However, this might contradict the traditional principle of autonomy as self-determination.

In the context of AI-based telemedicine for public health, autonomy ought to be rethought via a relational approach whereby individual autonomy can be promoted while acknowledging dependence on and responsibility of clinicians, public health experts, and legislators to drive patients' care. This would require enhancing patient trust and willingness to share data through public and patient engagement in research, instead of imposing legal obligations.

Justice and Fairness

Justice and fairness are commonly described in AI ethics as related to bias

BOX 1— Ethical Principles and Their Matched Themes for Artificial Intelligence (AI)-based Telemedicine for Public Health

Meaningful Ethical Principles for AI-Based Telemedicine for Public Health	Themes From AI Ethics Literature[17,19,29]	Themes From Bioethics, Medical Ethics, Telehealth, and Telemedicine Literature[33–36]	Themes From Public Health Ethics[37,38]
Benevolence and nonmaleficence	Ensure AI safety, accuracy, and efficacy Empower human beings Prevent or minimize AI's mental or physical harm to individuals and groups	Benefit patient welfare Improve access to quality and interruption-free health care Do not cause pain or suffering	Gear effectiveness and efficiency toward reducing morbidity and mortality Create least infringement and least necessity of public justification Use noncoerciveness
Autonomy: "Respect people's decision-making"	Ensure meaningful human oversight Protect privacy and confidentiality Avoid manipulation and experimentation without informed consent	Respect human self-determination and decision-making at individual and relational (communal attachments) levels Provide good professional–patient relationship (clinicians' confidentiality) and fidelity	Ensure connectedness and solidarity, liberty, and self-determination
Justice and Fairness: "Treat people fairly"	Ensure inclusiveness, absence of bias, and equity in AI systems' access, use, design, data, and outcomes	Treat persons fairly, equitably, and appropriately: employ distributive justice and sociorelational justice Provide fair and balanced access	Ensure participation of public and the affected parties: procedural justice Distribute burdens and benefits fairly
Explicability	For technology robustness, ensure AI transparency, resilience, security, accuracy, reliability, and reproducibility Ensure AI intelligibility	Tell the truth	Disclose information and speak truthfully: transparency Avoid paternalism
Responsibility and Accountability	Ensure human warranty and third-party regulatory bodies' approval Implement harm redress mechanisms Ensure responsibility and liability		Ensure communal responsibility and community cohesiveness Be responsible to minimize burden on populations
Sustainability and Responsiveness	Ensure AI promotes health and environmental and work sustainability Ensure health protection and promotion		Ensure sustainability of the global environment and human systems: precautionary principle Ensure cost effectiveness and usefulness

Note. The box presents a summary mapping of ethical themes from AI ethics, bioethics, medical ethics (telemedicine and telehealth), and public health ethics toward a unified set of revised AI ethics principles for AI-based telemedicine.

and discrimination in ML. Indeed, beyond risks caused by the digital health divide and literacy, there are risks of systematic iatrogenic harm to increase health injustice when algorithms are not trained on data that is representative of the population that they are intended to serve. In AI-based telemedicine for public health, the design of these systems ought to be centered on the most vulnerable and marginalized and be deployed with adequate consideration of such populations' needs and their ability to access and use them.[39]

Explicability

Public health interventions require consent of the population to be effective. To obtain consent, they must be intelligible to the public. AI-based telemedicine poses a challenge in public health considering that ML is often a black box. AI systems ought to meet the principle of explicability, which is not only a key safety mechanism but also an important public health principle to encourage widespread adoption.

Responsibility and Accountability

In the context of AI-based telemedicine, there are concerns about the need for responsibility and accountability once technologies are implemented. Existing regulatory systems are not designed to manage AI systems, which require continuous regulation during their life cycle and may consist of ever-changing algorithms. Furthermore, the problem of accountability is emphasized when AI is compared with other public health interventions, which often have close human oversight. Different teams may create, regulate, license, and operate AI solutions, which can make it ambiguous where liability lies. Thus, clear and understandable guidelines for responsibility distribution and harm redress mechanisms ought to be put in place.

Sustainability and Responsiveness

To be effective in the long term, AI-based telemedicine ought to be designed to evolve over time (i.e., to be sustainable) and adapt to the needs of a changing population (i.e., to be responsive). Data shifts over time present a challenge to AI, because changes in population characteristics may result in the algorithms being later operationalized for a population different from the one they were trained on. Also, to encourage adoption and trigger positive public response, there needs to be public trust in AI, which requires evidence of effectiveness, efficiency, and proportionality.

AN AI-BASED TELEMEDICINE APPLICATION

AiCure (AiCure, New York, NY) is a remote patient monitoring and management telemedicine tool. It consists of a mobile telephone application that uses facial analytics to aid medication adherence. To this aim, AiCure uses ML to analyze patients' videos to detect complete swallowing and the correct pill. AiCure might be described as compliant with the principle of benevolence insofar as it has been shown to benefit people in terms of accuracy and effectiveness. Indeed, in 2017, AiCure was demonstrated to be 25% better at ensuring drug adherence in schizophrenic patients than was a drug concentration measurement–based system.[40]

Although medication adherence appears to be on the surface a beneficent goal, this must be balanced with the consideration of patient autonomy. AiCure relies on automatic alerts sent to users, their relatives, friends, and physicians and HCPs to promote medication adherence. Hence, it could be argued that AiCure adopts a paternalistic approach to health care wherein repeated electronic notifications and users' fear of negative repercussions from third parties being notified of noncompliance nudge them into taking medication. Paternalistic approaches fail to consider users' personal circumstances and fluid preferences. For instance, patients may choose to forego medication for various rational reasons, including concerns about side effects and competing priorities with other aspects of life. From a public health perspective, the issue can be reframed based on the principle of proportionality: is the medication being monitored of sufficient importance to justify infringing patient autonomy?[27]

Such proportionality should factor in the medication's impact on patients (e.g., whether the medication is lifesaving) and on wider society. For instance, antibiotic medication may not be perceived as necessary for life, but nonadherence may cause society to suffer from the spread of infection. Consequently, respect for autonomy might need to be reconsidered via a relational lens, as acknowledged in bioethics, medical ethics, and public health ethics, in which the promotion of individual autonomy cannot prescind from the protection of the community and in which autonomy more than self-determination requires solidarity.

Privacy and confidentiality are widely considered in the ethical frameworks as 2 key requirements for the respect for autonomy. Health-monitoring devices collect vast amounts of users' personal information. AiCure gathers images and videos used for assessing medication adherence, including users' biometric, voice recording, and Internet traffic data.[27] This raises the question of whether patients retain the legal right to control these data. Maintaining patients' trust and respect requires at least providing them with intelligible information on what is being done with their data and who can access it (i.e., explicability), the possibility to grant or rescind permission to specific bodies, and the means to withdraw any collected data (i.e., meaningful control and oversight). In addition, whether patients remain owners of personal health data that have been de-identified depends on the jurisdiction in which the data were collected and the local data governance laws. In the case of AiCure, the use of facial analytics raises the concern that even anonymized patient data could be de-anonymized without much difficulty. Hence, a careful balancing of patients' rights and technological advancement for health optimization is needed with regard to data ownership.

Data confidentiality poses another ethical consideration. An important feature of AiCure is the ability to share patient data with clinicians, friends, and family members. Although clinicians are governed by strict confidentiality regulations, friends and family typically are not. Thus, some have questioned whether such individuals should be required to undertake duties of patient confidentiality akin to clinicians. In this case, for example, revising the ethical principle of autonomy via a relational approach might entail considering how to extend ethical duties of confidentiality to patients' core social relations.

From the perspective of justice and fairness, although AiCure can promote justice by providing a service for hard-to-reach groups, access is restricted to those who possess and are sufficiently competent with smartphones that have camera capability. Also, AiCure's efficacy is restricted to people that have friends, relatives, and HCPs with the means to receive remote electronic notifications and the knowledge to act on the information provided. This raises concerns about equal access to opportunities for certain groups, including those who are more isolated, socially deprived, and less technologically or health literate. Moreover, the exclusion of certain groups in the design and use of AI technologies can introduce bias into data sets and lead ML to produce erroneous health outputs for users belonging to excluded groups. From a public health perspective, this could negatively influence public trust and willingness to engage with not only the application directly involved in such errors but also similar technologies, which can contribute to the continued exclusion of certain groups. Therefore, it is crucial to ensure equity in user representation with specific attention to the inclusion of marginalized and vulnerable groups in deploying designs and tests and using AI-assisted telemedicine tools.

The analysis of a real-world AI-based telemedicine application through a few of the lenses of our ethical framework shows the value of such principles in highlighting a range of complex ethical considerations and risks that would otherwise be difficult to detect. Such risks, if unaddressed, can lead to adopting tools that, rather than promoting, can undermine individuals' rights and public health. The considerations highlighted also show the need to further work and refine, via the analyses of case studies, the ethical principles we propose to render them adequate in accounting for trade-off scenarios and provide more actionable guidelines on how to overcome them.

CONCLUSIONS

We have argued that AI-based telemedicine has the potential to be a strong aid to public health ecosystems worldwide by enabling better clinical health and care, from health monitoring to disease prevention and management, at both the individual and population levels. However, AI-based telemedicine can also present specific ethical risks that can harm individuals and counteract public health goals, such as the promotion of better health care and health equity. The absence of a context-sensitive ethical framework to assess such technology hampers the detection of ethical risks, jeopardizing the potential of AI-based telemedicine for public health. Indeed, some of the risks we have highlighted, such as improper data sharing and discrimination, might undermine people's trust in AI-based telemedicine and make public health actors reluctant to adopt such tools, leading to a potential opportunity loss.

We have tried to demonstrate the importance of mapping and revising current AI ethics principles for AI-based telemedicine for public health. To do so, we have considered prominent ethical frameworks underpinning the main domains such technology intersects to revise general ethics frameworks developed for the use of AI broadly and for health specifically. Without pretending to be exhaustive, we hope that our framework can offer an ethical compass for those who design and implement such systems in and for public health. Furthermore, we hope that our effort in highlighting relevant ethical principles for AI-based telemedicine will spur further conceptual and technical research to better refine and operationalize such principles to render AI-based telemedicine a true force for public health. AJPH

ABOUT THE AUTHORS

Simona Tiribelli is with the Department of Political Sciences, Communication, and International Relations, University of Macerata, Macerata, Italy, and the Institute for Technology and Global Health, Cambridge, MA. Annabelle Monnot is with Polygeia, Global Health Think Tank, Cambridge, UK. Syed F. H. Shah and Anmol Arora are with the School of Clinical Medicine, University of Cambridge, Cambridge. Ping J. Toong is with the Department of Pathology, University of Cambridge. Sokanha Kong is with the Department of Medical Genetics, University of Cambridge.

CORRESPONDENCE

Correspondence should be sent to Simona Tiribelli, Don Giovanni Minzoni, 22/A, 62100 Macerata MC, Italy (e-mail: simona.tiribelli@unimc.it). Reprints can be ordered at http://www.ajph.org by clicking the "Reprints" link.

PUBLICATION INFORMATION

Full Citation: Tiribelli S, Monnot A, Shah SFH, Arora A, Toong PJ, Kong S. Ethics principles for artificial intelligence–based telemedicine for public health. *Am J Public Health*. 2023;113(5):577–584.

Acceptance Date: January 2, 2023.

DOI: https://doi.org/10.2105/AJPH.2023.307225

CONTRIBUTORS

S. Tiribelli defined the research thesis, the study concept, and the structure of the article and contributed substantially to the writing and editing. A. Monnot synthetized the analyses and led the writing of the first draft of the article. S. F. H. Shah, A. Arora, P. J. Toong, and S. Kong assisted with the research and writing. All authors conceptualized ideas, interpreted findings, and reviewed drafts of the article.

ACKNOWLEDGMENTS

We would like to thank the 2021 Polygeia Cambridge Committee for providing the framework under which this collaboration with the Institute for Technology and Global Health in the project AI Ethics for AI-Based Telemedicine led by S. Tiribelli occurred.

CONFLICTS OF INTEREST

The authors have no conflicts of interest to declare.

HUMAN PARTICIPANT PROTECTION

No protocol approval was necessary because no human participants were involved in this study.

REFERENCES

1. Centers for Disease Control and Prevention. Telehealth and telemedicine: a research anthology of law and policy resources. July 26, 2019. Available at: https://www.cdc.gov/phlp/publications/topic/anthologies/anthologies-telehealth.html. Accessed October 28, 2022.
2. Raheja A, Manjunath N, Garg K, et al. Turning a new chapter in neurosurgery outpatient services: telemedicine a "savior" in this pandemic. *Neurol India*. 2021;69(2):344–351. https://doi.org/10.4103/0028-3886.31452
3. Cabieses B, Faba G, Espinoza M, Santorelli G. The link between information and communication technologies and global public health: pushing forward. *Telemed J E Health*. 2013;19(11):879–87. https://doi.org/10.1089/tmj.2012.0232
4. Jones LD, Golan D, Hanna SA, Ramachandran M. Artificial intelligence, machine learning and the evolution of healthcare: a bright future or cause for concern? *Bone Joint Res*. 2018;7(3):223–225. https://doi.org/10.1302/2046-3758.73.BJR-2017-0147.R1
5. Nevin L; PLOS Medicine Editors. Advancing the beneficial use of machine learning in health care and medicine: toward a community understanding. *PLoS Med*. 2018;15(11):e1002708. https://doi.org/10.1371/journal.pmed.1002708
6. Darkins AW, Cary MA. *Telemedicine and Telehealth: Principles, Policies, Performances and Pitfalls*. New York, NY: Springer; 2000.
7. Bashshur R, Shannon G, Krupinski E, Grigsby J. The taxonomy of telemedicine. *Telemed J E Health*. 2011;17(6):484–494. https://doi.org/10.1089/tmj.2011.0103
8. Doarn CR, Merrell RC. Telemedicine, telehealth, and the public health good. *Telemed J E Health*. 2019;25(9):773–774. https://doi.org/10.1089/tmj.2019.29028.crd
9. Khoury MJ, Iademarco MF, Riley WT. Precision public health for the era of precision medicine. *Am J Prev Med*. 2016;50(3):398–401. https://doi.org/10.1016/j.amepre.2015.08.031
10. Kuziemsky C, Maeder AJ, John O, et al. Role of artificial intelligence within the telehealth domain. *Yearb Med Inform*. 2019;28(1):35–40. https://doi.org/10.1055/s-0039-1677897
11. Byerly S, Maurer LR, Mantero A, Naar L, An G, Kaafarani HMA. Machine learning and artificial intelligence for surgical decision making. *Surg Infect (Larchmt)*. 2021;22(6):626–634. https://doi.org/10.1089/sur.2021.007
12. Rasmussen SA, Khoury MJ, Del Rio C. Precision public health as a key tool in the COVID-19 response. *JAMA*. 2020;324(10):933–934. https://doi.org/10.1001/jama.2020.14992
13. Singh H. Using analytics for better decision-making. December 1, 2018. Available at: https://towardsdatascience.com/using-analytics-for-better-decision-making-ce4f92c4a025. Accessed November 1, 2022.
14. Bhaskar S, Bradley S, Sakhamuri S, et al. Designing futuristic telemedicine using artificial intelligence and robotics in the COVID-19 era. *Front Public Health*. 2020;8:556789. https://doi.org/10.3389/fpubh.2020.556789
15. Adamson AS, Smith A. Machine learning and health care disparities in dermatology. *JAMA Dermatol*. 2018;154(11):1247–1248. https://doi.org/10.1001/jamadermatol.2018.2348
16. Kakani P, Chandra A, Mullainathan S, Obermeyer Z. Allocation of COVID-19 relief funding to disproportionately Black counties. *JAMA*. 2020;324(10):1000–1003. https://doi.org/10.1001/jama.2020.14978
17. European Commission, Directorate-General for Communications Networks, Content and Technology. Ethics guidelines for trustworthy AI. 2019. Available at: https://data.europa.eu/doi/10.2759/346720. Available at: https://op.europa.eu/en/publication-detail/-/publication/d3988569-0434-11ea-8c1f-01aa75ed71a1. Accessed August 8, 2022.
18. US Food and Drug Administration. Artificial intelligence/machine learning (AI/ML)–based software as a medical device (SaMD) action plan. September 22, 2021. Available at: https://www.fda.gov/medical-devices/software-medical-device-samd/artificial-intelligence-and-machine-learning-software-medical-device. Accessed January 22, 2023.
19. World Health Organization. Ethics and governance of artificial intelligence for health. June 28, 2021. Available at: https://www.who.int/publications/i/item/9789240029200. Accessed May 9, 2022.
20. Bhattacharya S, Hossain MM, Juyal R, Sharma N, Pradhan KB, Singh A. Role of public health ethics for responsible use of artificial intelligence technologies. *Indian J Community Med*. 2021;46(2):178–181. https://doi.org/10.4103/ijcm.IJCM_62_20
21. Thomasian NM, Eickhoff C, Adashi EY. Advancing health equity with artificial intelligence. *J Public Health Policy*. 2021;42(4):602–611. https://doi.org/10.1057/s41271-021-00319-5
22. Khoury MJ, Ioannidis JP. Medicine. Big data meets public health. *Science*. 2014;346(6213):1054–1055. https://doi.org/10.1126/science.aaa2709
23. US Food and Drug Administration. Clinical decision support software: guidance for industry and Food and Drug Administration staff. May 6, 2020. Available at: https://www.fda.gov/regulatory-information/search-fda-guidance-documents/clinical-decision-support-software. Accessed May 9, 2022.
24. Chen J, See KC. Artificial intelligence for COVID-19: rapid review. *J Med Internet Res*. 2020;22(10):e21476. https://doi.org/10.2196/21476
25. Li J-PO, Liu H, Ting DSJ, et al. Digital technology, tele-medicine and artificial intelligence in ophthalmology: a global perspective. *Prog Retin Eye Res*. 2021;82:100900. https://doi.org/10.1016/j.preteyeres.2020.100900
26. Marchiori C, Dykeman D, Girardi I, et al. Artificial intelligence decision support for medical triage. *AMIA Annu Symp Proc*. 2021;2020:793–802.
27. Van Biesen W, Decruyenaere J, Sideri K, Cockbain J, Sterckx S. Remote digital monitoring of medication intake: methodological, medical, ethical and legal reflections. *Acta Clin Belg*. 2021;76(3):209–216. https://doi.org/10.1080/17843286.2019.1708152
28. Schrader L, Vargas Toro A, Konietzny S, et al. Advanced sensing and human activity recognition in early intervention and rehabilitation of elderly people. *J Popul Ageing*. 2020;13(2):139–165. https://doi.org/10.1007/s12062-020-09260-z
29. Jobin A, Ienca M, Vayena E. The global landscape of AI ethics guidelines. *Nat Mach Intell*. 2019;1(9):389–399. https://doi.org/10.1038/s42256-019-0088-2
30. American Telemedicine Association. The ethics and regulations of AI. April 15, 2019. Available at: https://www.americantelemed.org/resources/the-ethics-and-regulations-of-ai. Accessed November 10, 2022.
31. World Medical Association. WMA statement on the ethics of telemedicine. October 11, 2022. Available at: https://www.wma.net/policies-post/wma-statement-on-the-ethics-of-telemedicine. Accessed November 10, 2022.
32. American Medical Association. Ethical practice in telemedicine. Available at: https://www.ama-assn.org/delivering-care/ethics/ethical-practice-telemedicine. Accessed May 9, 2022.
33. Solomonides AE, Koski E, Atabaki SM, et al. Defining AMIA's artificial intelligence principles. *J Am Med Inform Assoc*. 2022;29(4):585–591. https://doi.org/10.1093/jamia/ocac006
34. Varkey B. Principles of clinical ethics and their application to practice. *Med Princ Pract*. 2021;30(1):17–28. https://doi.org/10.1159/000509119
35. Keenan AJ, Tsourtos G, Tieman J. The value of applying ethical principles in telehealth practices: systematic review. *J Med Internet Res*. 2021;23(3):e25698. https://doi.org/10.2196/25698
36. Fletcher J. Principles of biomedical ethics. *By Tom L. Beauchamp and James F. Childress*. New York, Oxford University Press, 1979. 314 pp. 13.95. 7.95 (paper). *Theol Today*. 1980;36(4):595–596. https://doi.org/10.1177/004057368003600423
37. Kass NE. An ethics framework for public health. *Am J Public Health*. 2001;91(11):1776–1782. https://doi.org/10.2105/AJPH.91.11.1776
38. Coughlin SS. How many principles for public health ethics? *Open Public Health J*. 2008;1:8–16. https://doi.org/10.2174/1874944500801010008
39. Giovanola B, Tiribelli S. Beyond bias and discrimination: redefining the AI ethics principle of fairness in healthcare machine-learning algorithms. *AI Soc*. 2022; Epub ahead of print. https://doi.org/10.1007/s00146-022-01455-6
40. Bain EE, Shafner L, Walling DP, et al. Use of a novel artificial intelligence platform on mobile devices to assess dosing compliance in a phase 2 clinical trial in subjects with schizophrenia. *JMIR Mhealth Uhealth*. 2017;5(2):e18. https://doi.org/10.2196/mhealth.7030

Erratum In: "Living Alone and Suicide Risk in the United States, 2008–2019"

In: Olfson M, Cosgrove CM, Altekruse SF, Wall MM, Blanco C. Living alone and suicide risk in the United States, 2008–2019. *Am J Public Health*. 2022;112(12):1774–1782.

When originally published, a result was incorrectly reported. On p. 1776, column 2, the second sentence of the first paragraph of the "Results" section should read: "As compared with people who lived with others, those who lived alone were significantly older and were more likely to be female, to have White or Black race/ethnicity, to have a low income, to reside in more urban rather than the most rural areas, to own rather than rent their residence, and to have a functional disability."

This change does not affect the article's conclusions. AJPH

https://doi.org/10.2105/AJPH.2022.307080e

Erratum In: "SARS-CoV-2 Infection, Hospitalization, and Death in Vaccinated and Infected Individuals by Age Groups in Indiana, 2021–2022"

In: Tu W, Zhang P, Roberts A, et al. SARS-CoV-2 infection, hospitalization, and death in vaccinated and infected individuals by age groups in Indiana, 2021–2022. *Am J Public Health*. 2023;113(1):96–104.

When originally published, censoring was reported incorrectly in the article. On p. 98, column 2, the first full sentence should read: "Matched pairs were censored when an infected participant received a vaccination."

This change does not affect the article's conclusions. AJPH

https://doi.org/10.2105/AJPH.2022.307112e

Erratum In: *American Journal of Public Health*, Volume 113, Issue 2

In: *Am J Public Health*. 2023;113(2):129–240

A cover line on a recent cover was incorrect. On the cover of the February 2023 issue, the fifth cover line should read:

Also in this issue:
PEACE AND PUBLIC HEALTH
When Peace Is Threatened,
So Is Public Health,
pp. 132 and 146–159

https://doi.org/10.2105/AJPH.2023.307279

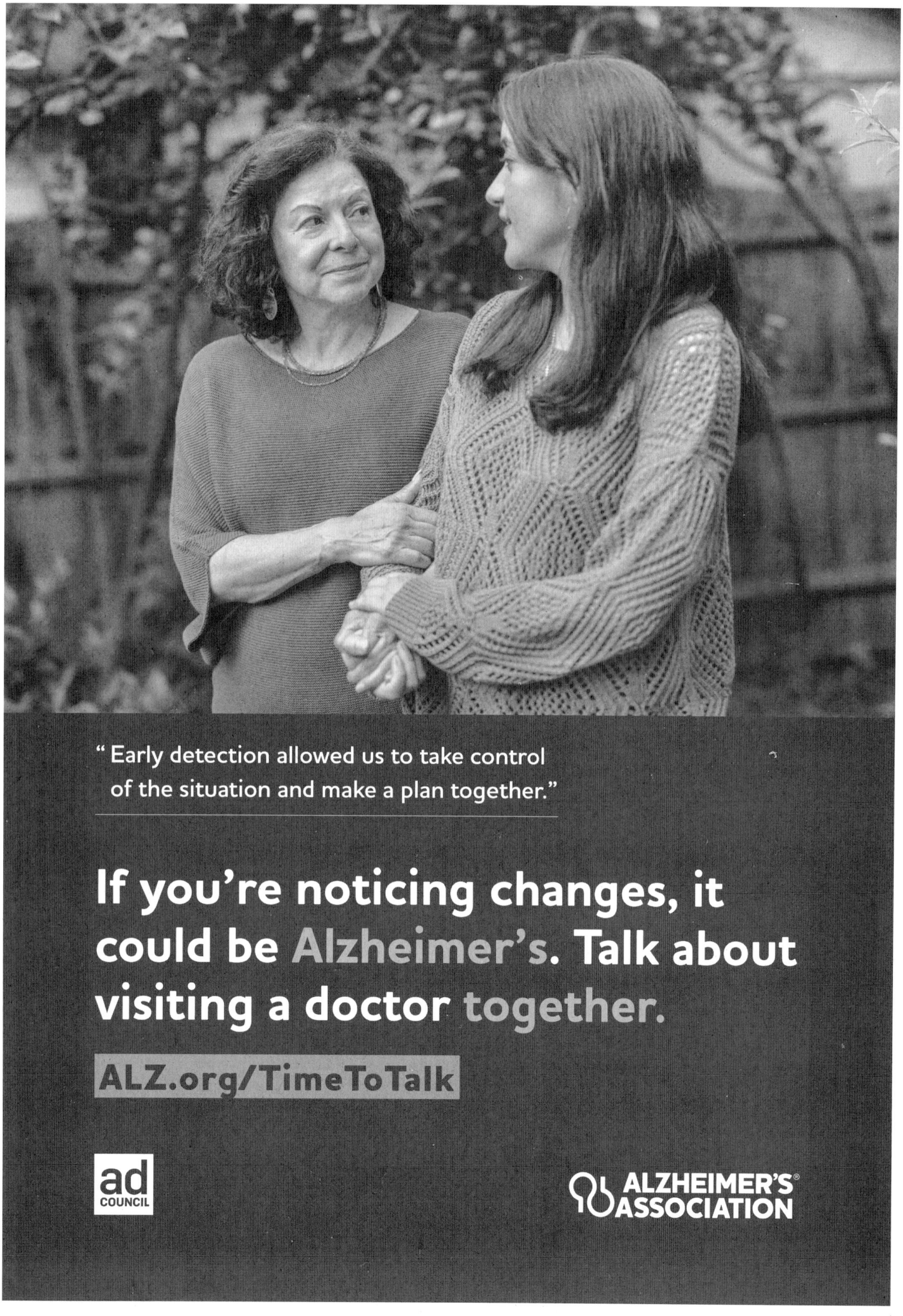

" Early detection allowed us to take control of the situation and make a plan together."
If you're noticing changes, it could be Alzheimer's. Talk about visiting a doctor together.
ALZ.org/TimeToTalk
ad COUNCIL
ALZHEIMER'S® ASSOCIATION

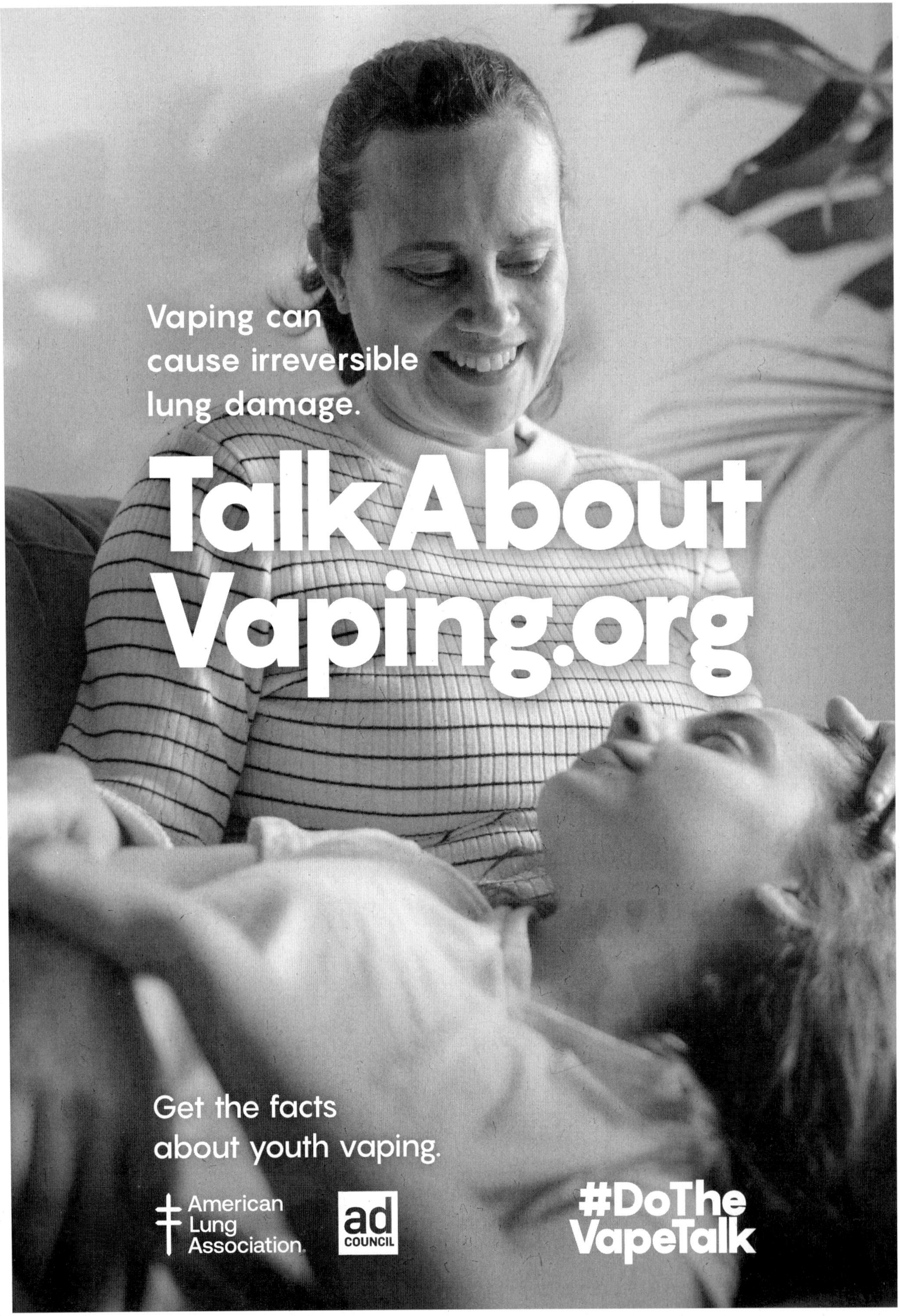

Vaping can
cause irreversible
lung damage.
TalkAbout
Vaping.org
Get the facts
about youth vaping.
American
Lung
Association.
ad
COUNCIL
#DoThe
VapeTalk